Worked Problems

in

Ophthalmic Lenses

by

A H Tunnacliffe and G D Janney

The Association of British Dispensing Opticians
College of Education
Godmersham Park
Godmersham
Canterbury
Kent
England
CT4 7DT

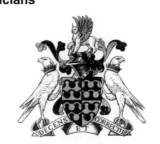

ISBN 0 - 900099 178

First Edition 1979
Reprinted in 1983 and 1987
Second Edition 1991
Third Edition 1997
Reprinted in 2005

Association of British Dispensing Opticians Publications

Optics	A. H. Tunnacliffe & J. G. Hirst
Introduction to Visual Optics 4th Edition	A. H. Tunnacliffe
The Principles of Ophthalmic Lenses	M. Jalie
Worked Problems in Optics	A. H. Tunnacliffe
Worked Problems in Ophthalmic Lenses	A. H. Tunnacliffe & G. D. Janney
Ocular Anatomy and Histology	D. M. Pipe & L. J. Rapley
Essentials of Dispensing	A. H. Tunnacliffe

Preface

In optometry and ophthalmic dispensing, a large proportion of the examination questions in ophthalmic lenses consists of mathematically based problems. The author believes a student must spend considerable time in learning to solve such problems. The effort is not inconsiderable. However, the reward gained is a deeper understanding of the theory and an an increased facility for tackling problems.

There is a well established supply of worked problems books for students of mathematics and the sciences, but there is a dearth of this genre for opticians and optometrists. In general, text books do not have sufficient space for a great number of worked examples. In this context, the present text is to be regarded as a supplement to a main text.

After studying the theory the student should try relevant questions from this book. If the problem can be completed then the answer confirms the student's grasp of the subject. If, however, the student cannot start or complete a problem then the answer can be used to overcome the difficulty. The student should not treat these worked problems as examples simply to be read. He/she must struggle with the question and only use the answer when a hint or a confirmation is required. The second time around, however, the answers may prove useful for revision.

There is a companion volume dealing with optics problems. Again the book parallels the usual treatment of the subject in a main text. Both worked problems books have been updated with new questions.

Bradford   A H Tunnacliffe
                                                               G D Janney

June 1997

The Greek Alphabet

A number of symbols from the Greek alphabet are used in the text.   For convenience the whole alphabet is given below, together with each letter's name.

A	α	alpha
B	β	beta
Γ	γ	gamma
Δ	δ	delta
E	ε	epsilon
Z	ζ	zeta
H	η	eta
Θ	θ	theta
I	ι	iota
K	κ	kappa
Λ	λ	lambda
M	μ	mu
N	ν	nu
Ξ	ξ	xi
O	ο	omicron
Π	π	pi
P	ρ	rho
Σ	σ	sigma
T	τ	tau
Y	υ	upsilon
Ψ	ψ	psi
Ω	ω	omega

Contents

1	BACKGROUND OPTICAL PRINCIPLES	1
2	THIN LENS AND SURFACE POWER	2
3	CYLINDRICAL AND SPHERO-CYLINDRICAL LENSES	6
4	THE LENS MEASURE, SAG AND THICKNESS	19
5	OPHTHALMIC PRISMS	36
6	PRISMATIC EFFECTS	52
7	MINIMUM SIZE OF UNCUT AND FIELD OF VIEW	90
8	BIFOCALS AND TRIFOCALS	96
9	PROTECTIVE LENSES	115
10	OBLIQUELY CROSSED CYLINDERS	128
11	LENS FORM AND EFFECTIVITY	137
12	BEST FORM LENSES	142

1   BACKGROUND OPTICAL PRINCIPLES

1   **Define the following:**
   (a) **Optical or principal axis.**   (b) **Front and back vertices.**
   (c) **Radius of curvature.**   (d) **Optical centre.**

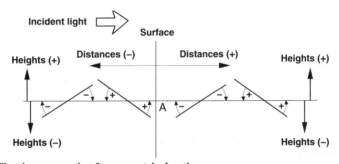

Refer to figure 1.1.

(a) The optical axis of a lens is an imaginary straight line passing through the centres of curvature, C_1 and C_2, of the two surfaces.

(b) The front and back vertices are the points at which the optical axis intersects the front and back surfaces of the lens, respectively. See the points A_1 and A_2.

(c) The radius of curvature of a surface is the distance from that surface to its centre of curvature. For example, $r_2 = A_2C_2$ for the back surface, or $r_1 = A_1C_1$ for the front surface.

(d) The optical centre, O, is a point lying on the optical axis such that a ray passing through this point is undeviated.

---

2   **With the aid of a diagram, describe the sign convention used in geometrical optics.**

Fig. 1.2   The sign convention for geometrical optics.

(a) Light is assumed to travel from left to right.
(b) Measurement of a distance along the axis is taken from the thin lens or surface.
(c) Measurements taken in the same direction as the incident light is travelling are positive. Those taken in the opposite direction are negative.
(d) A measurement from the otpical axis to a point above it is positive, and to a point below is negative.
(e) Angles measured in an anticlockwise direction are positive, and those in a clockwise direction are negative.
(f) Angles between the ray and the optical axis are measured from the ray to the axis.
(g) The angle of incidence or refraction at a surface is measured from the normal to the ray.

2   THIN LENS AND SURFACE POWER

1   **Find the power in dioptres of the lenses whose focal lengths are:**
    (i) +25 cm   **(ii) −129 mm**   **(iii) +80 cm**   **(iv) −4000 mm.**

Note: the focal length is taken to be the second focal length, f', so that for a thin lens in air the power is $F = 1/f'$, where f' is in metres.

(i) $F = \dfrac{1}{f'} = \dfrac{1}{+0.25} = +4.00 \text{ D}$ (ii) $F = \dfrac{1}{f'} = \dfrac{1}{-0.129} = -7.75 \text{ D}$

(iii) $F = \dfrac{1}{f'} = \dfrac{1}{+0.80} = +1.25 \text{ D}$ (iv) $F = \dfrac{1}{f'} = \dfrac{1}{-4.000} = -0.25 \text{ D}$

---

2   **Find the focal lengths, expressed in centimetres, of the following lenses whose powers are:**   **(i) +2.25 D,**   **(ii) −0.75 D,**   **(iii) +13.25 D,**   **(iv) −9.50 D.**

Again, assume the lens to be thin and in air, and the focal length required to be the second focal length f'.

(i) $f' = \dfrac{1}{F} = \dfrac{1}{+2.25} = +0.4444 \text{ m} = +44.44 \text{ cm.}$

(ii) $f' = \dfrac{1}{F} = \dfrac{1}{-0.75} = -1.3333 \text{ m} = -133.33 \text{ cm.}$

(iii) $f' = \dfrac{1}{F} = \dfrac{1}{+13.25} = +0.07547 \text{ m} = +7.547 \text{ cm.}$

(iv) $f' = \dfrac{1}{F} = \dfrac{1}{-9.5} = -0.1053 \text{ m} = -10.53 \text{ cm.}$

---

3   **Spherical surfaces of the following radii are worked on glass of refractive index 1.523. Find the power of each surface.**
    (i) +26.15 mm **(ii) +13.075 cm** **(iii) −52.3 cm** **(iv) −100 mm.**

The power of each surface will be given in dioptres when the radius is in metres in the equation $F = \dfrac{n' - n}{r}$.

(i) $F = \dfrac{n' - n}{r} = \dfrac{1.523 - 1}{+0.02615} = +20.00 \text{ D}$ (ii) $F = \dfrac{n' - n}{r} = \dfrac{1.523 - 1}{+0.13075} = +4.00 \text{ D}$

(iii) $F = \dfrac{n' - n}{r} = \dfrac{1.523 - 1}{-0.523} = -1.00 \text{ D}$ (iv) $F = \dfrac{n' - n}{r} = \dfrac{1.523 - 1}{-0.100} = -5.23 \text{ D.}$

4 The radii of the surfaces of a number of thin lenses are as follows. Find the power of the lenses if $n = 1.52$.
(a) $r_1 = +86.67$ mm, $r_2 = +173.33$ mm   (b) $r_1 = +23.11$ cm, $r_2 = +8.32$ cm
(c) $r_1 = +130$ mm, $r_2 = -260$ mm.

We use the surface power relationship to obtain the power of each surface in turn, adhering strictly to the sign convention.

(a) $F_1 = \dfrac{n_1' - n_1}{r_1} = \dfrac{1.52 - 1}{+0.08667} = +6.00$ D   and $F_2 = \dfrac{n_2' - n_2}{r_2} = \dfrac{1 - 1.52}{+0.17333} = -3.00$ D.

The *thin* lens power is given by $F = F_1 + F_2 = (+6.00) + (-3.00) = +3.00$ D.

(b) $F_1 = \dfrac{n_1' - n_1}{r_1} = \dfrac{1.52 - 1}{+0.2311} = +2.25$ D   and $F_2 = \dfrac{n_2' - n_2}{r_2} = \dfrac{1 - 1.52}{+0.0832} = -6.25$ D.

Hence, the lens power is $F = F_1 + F_2 = (+2.25) + (-6.25) = -4.00$ D.

(c) $F_1 = \dfrac{n_1' - n_1}{r_1} = \dfrac{1.52 - 1}{+0.130} = +4.00$ D   and $F_2 = \dfrac{n_2' - n_2}{r_2} = \dfrac{1 - 1.52}{-0.260} = +2.00$ D.

Hence, the lens power is $F = F_1 + F_2 = (+4.00) + (+2.00) = +6.00$ D.

---

5 Calculate the radii of curvature in mm of each surface of the following thin lenses made from glass of refractive index 1.523.
(a) +3.50 D equiconvex   (b) –1.50 D meniscus (+6.00 D base)
(c) +2.50 D meniscus (+7.50 D base).

(a) Since the form of the lens is equiconvex, then $F_1 = F_2 = \dfrac{F}{2} = \dfrac{+3.50}{2} = +1.75$ D.

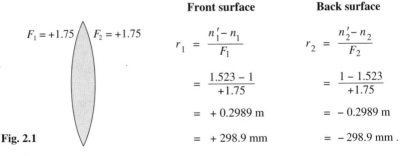

	Front surface	Back surface
$F_1 = +1.75$ $F_2 = +1.75$	$r_1 = \dfrac{n_1' - n_1}{F_1}$	$r_2 = \dfrac{n_2' - n_2}{F_2}$
	$= \dfrac{1.523 - 1}{+1.75}$	$= \dfrac{1 - 1.523}{+1.75}$
	$= +0.2989$ m	$= -0.2989$ m
Fig. 2.1	$= +298.9$ mm	$= -298.9$ mm .

(b) F_1 and F are given, so $F_2 = F - F_1 = (-1.50) - (+6.00) = -7.50$ D.

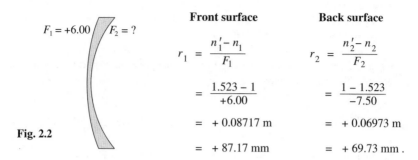

$F_1 = +6.00$ $F_2 = ?$

Front surface

$$r_1 = \frac{n_1' - n_1}{F_1}$$

$$= \frac{1.523 - 1}{+6.00}$$

$$= +0.08717 \text{ m}$$

$$= +87.17 \text{ mm}$$

Fig. 2.2

Back surface

$$r_2 = \frac{n_2' - n_2}{F_2}$$

$$= \frac{1 - 1.523}{-7.50}$$

$$= +0.06973 \text{ m}$$

$$= +69.73 \text{ mm .}$$

(c) F_1 and F are given, so $F_2 = F - F_1 = (+2.50) - (+7.50) = -5.00$ D.

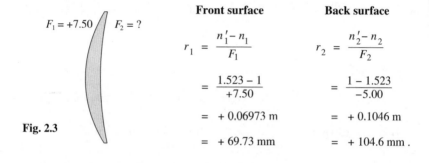

$F_1 = +7.50$ $F_2 = ?$

Front surface

$$r_1 = \frac{n_1' - n_1}{F_1}$$

$$= \frac{1.523 - 1}{+7.50}$$

$$= +0.06973 \text{ m}$$

$$= +69.73 \text{ mm}$$

Fig. 2.3

Back surface

$$r_2 = \frac{n_2' - n_2}{F_2}$$

$$= \frac{1 - 1.523}{-5.00}$$

$$= +0.1046 \text{ m}$$

$$= +104.6 \text{ mm .}$$

---

6   **It is required to produce a lens with surface powers +6.25 DS and –1.25 DS in glass of refractive index 1.654 . The prescription house only has surfacing tools for use with glass of refractive index 1.523 . Which tools must be used?**

Let T be the tool power and F the desired surface power. n_g is the refractive index of the glass actually being used and n_t is the refractive index for which the tool is calibrated.

Method   (i) Calculate the radius of curvature of the surface which will produce the required power in the glass which is to be used. That is,

$$r_1 = \frac{n_1' - n_1}{F_1} = \frac{n_g - 1}{F_1} \quad \text{for the front surface} \quad — \quad equation\ (1)$$

$$\text{and } r_2 = \frac{n_2' - n_2}{F_2} = \frac{1 - n_g}{F_2} \quad \text{for the back surface} \quad — \quad equation\ (2)$$

(ii) Using these radii of curvature, calculate the powers required using the refractive index for which the tools are marked. That is,

$$T_1 = \frac{n_t - 1}{r_1} \quad \text{for the front surface and } \quad T_2 = \frac{1 - n_t}{r_2} \quad \text{for the back surface.}$$

4

Front surface $r_1 = \dfrac{n_1' - n_1}{F_1} = \dfrac{n_g - 1}{F_1} = \dfrac{1.654 - 1}{+6.25} = +0.10464$ m

and $T_1 = \dfrac{n_t - 1}{r_1} = \dfrac{1.523 - 1}{+0.10464} = +4.99$ D $\approx +5.00$ D.

Back surface $r_2 = \dfrac{n_2' - n_2}{F_2} = \dfrac{1 - n_g}{F_2} = \dfrac{1 - 1.654}{-1.25} = +0.5232$ m

and $T_2 = \dfrac{1 - n_t}{r_2} = \dfrac{1 - 1.523}{+0.5232} = -0.9996$ D ≈ -1.00 D.

It should be noted that the two stage operation can be condensed by substituting for r from equation (1) into equation (2) to give an expression for T. That is,

$$T = \left(\frac{n_t - 1}{n_g - 1}\right) F.$$

---

7 **A −10.00 D lens is to be made from glass of refractive index 1.654, but the surface tools available have been made for use with glass of refractive index 1.523. A tool marked +3.00 D is used for the front surface. Which spectacle tool must be used for the back surface?**

Find the radius of curvature of the surface which has been worked on the front surface of the lens:

$$r_1 = \frac{n_1' - n_1}{F_1} = \frac{1.523 - 1}{+3.00} = +0.1743 \text{ m}.$$

Find the actual power which has been worked on the front surface of the lens:

$$F_1 = \frac{n_1' - n_1}{r_1} = \frac{1.654 - 1}{+0.1743} = +3.75 \text{ D}.$$

Find the power to be provided by the back surface:

$$F_2 = F - F_1 = (-10) - (+3.75) = -13.75 \text{ D}.$$

Find the radius of curvature of F_2 in glass of refractive index 1.654:

$$r_2 = \frac{n_2' - n_2}{F_2} = \frac{1 - 1.654}{-13.75} = +0.04756 \text{ m}.$$

Find the tool required using the above radius of curvature:

$$F_2 = \frac{n_2' - n_2}{r_2} = \frac{1 - 1.654}{+0.04756} = -10.99 \text{ D} \approx -11.00 \text{ D}.$$

---

3 CYLINDRICAL AND SPHERO-CYLINDRICAL LENSES

1 Use power diagrams (optical crosses) to find the principal powers of the thin flat lens +5.00 DS / +2.00 DC x 90 .

The spherical power will be worked on one surface and the cylindrical power on the other. From the thin lens equation $F = F_1 + F_2$ it is evident that the sum of the two surface powers is equal to the lens power. Noting that there is zero power along the axis meridian of the cylindrical surface and applying the thin lens equation in power diagram form below, with the sphere power on one surface and the cyl power on the other, we have the results shown in figure 3.1 .

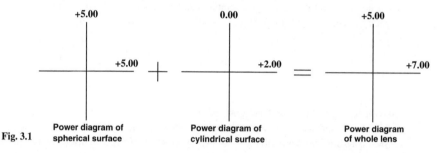

Fig. 3.1   Power diagram of spherical surface   Power diagram of cylindrical surface   Power diagram of whole lens

Therefore, the principal powers of the lens are +5.00 D along 90° and +7.00 D along 180°.

---

2 State the prescription, in sphero-cylindrical form, of the lens which has the following principal powers: **+1.75 D along 90° and +0.50 D along 180°.**

The principal powers of any sphero-cylindrical lens consist of one meridian containing the power of the *sphere* and the other meridian containing the power of the *sphere + cyl*.
Draw a power diagram of the lens: see figure 3.2 .

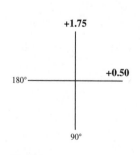

Fig. 3.2

Let the lower powered meridian be the sphere power (*S*). That is, + 0.50 DS. To obtain the cylinder power, subtract the lower powered meridian from the higher powered meridian: in symbols, using *S* for sphere power and *C* for cyl power,

$$(S + C) - S = C,$$

and in numbers

$$(+1.75) - (+0.50) = +1.25\,\text{DC}.$$

The axis is the meridian in which the cylinder has no power; that is, 180°. Hence, written in the sph/cyl form the prescription is +0.50 DS / +1.25 DC x 180.

Check Draw a power diagram of each element in the sph/cyl form and add them together. That is,

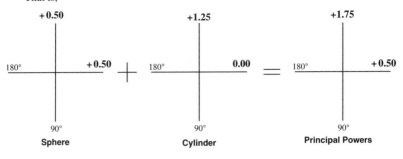

Fig. 3.3   The power diagram represented in sph / cyl form.

---

3   **Transpose the lens −2.75 DS / −0.50 DC x 45 into its alternate sphero-cylindrical form.**

(a) From the solution to question 3.2, it is clear that either principal meridian may be considered to contain the power of the *sphere*, and likewise, either can contain the power of the *sphere + cyl*. Therefore, to find the alternate sphero-cylindrical form from first principles, it is necessary to determine the principal powers. This is shown in figure 3.4 where the sphere and cylinder powers are added in power diagrams.

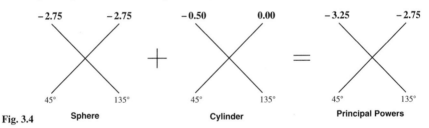

Fig. 3.4   Sphere   Cylinder   Principal Powers

If the meridian with power −3.25 D is now taken to be the sphere, then the cyl power will be obtained from $C = (S + C) - S = (-2.75) - (-3.25) = +0.50$ DC, the axis in this case being 135°. Note that S and C stand for the sphere and cylinder powers and the cyl axis lies along the S meridian.

The alternate sph/cyl form is therefore −3.25 DS / + 0.50 DC x 135.

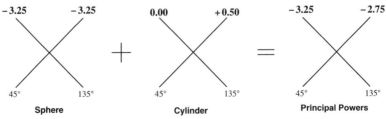

Fig. 3.5   Addition of power diagrams of the alternate sph/cyl form gives the same lens power as in figure 3.4.

(b) Transposition of this lens into its alternate sph/cyl form may also be accomplished by following the rules with which the reader is assumed to be familiar.
   (i)   Add algebraically the sphere and the cylinder to obtain the new sphere:
         $$(-2.75) + (-0.50) = -3.25 \text{ DS}$$
   (ii) Change the sign of the cylinder $\Rightarrow$ +0.50 DC.
   (iii) Change the cyl axis through 90° $\Rightarrow$ 135°.

That is, -3.25 DS $/ + 0.50$ DC x 135.

---

4   Transpose each of the following prescriptions into its crossed cylinder form:
   (a)   +1.50 DS / +2.75 DC x 180   **(b)   −1.50 DS / +1.00 DC x 135**
   (c)   +1.75 DS / −4.25 DC x 60.

(a)

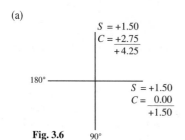

Fig. 3.6

Draw a power diagram, combining the sphere and the cylinder onto one optical cross:

See figure 3.6.

This gives a +1.50 D cylinder with its axis at 90°, and a +4.25 D cylinder with its axis at 180°. That is, the crossed cylinder form is

$$+1.50 \text{ DC x } 90 / +4.25 \text{ DC x } 180.$$

(b)

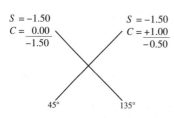

Fig. 3.7

Adopting the same procedure we have, from figure 3.7, the crossed cylinder form as:

$$-0.50 \text{ DC x } 135 / -1.50 \text{ DC x } 45 .$$

(c)

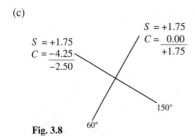

Fig. 3.8

Again, we draw the power diagram; see figure 3.8.

The crossed cylinder form is

$$+1.75 \text{ DC x } 150 / -2.50 \text{ DC x } 60 .$$

5 **What is the sphero / cylindrical equivalent of each of the following crossed cyls?**
(a) **+1.25 DC x 90 / +3.25 DC x 180**   **(b)** **−0.75 DC x 60 / −1.25 DC x 150**
(c) **−1.00 DC x 135 / +1.50 DC x 45** .

As before, in any sph / cyl lens, either principal meridian may be considered to contain the power of the *sphere*, or the power of the *sphere + cyl*. This simply means the same power can be made in the two alternate sph / cyl forms. We shall arbitrarily take the numerically lower power to be the power of the sphere.

(a) Draw a power diagram; see figure 3.9 .

In this case then, the horizontal meridian contains the sphere power, that is +1.25 D, and the power of the cylinder is therefore

$$C = (S + C) - S$$
$$= (+3.25) - (+1.25) = +2.00 \text{ D.}$$

The axis is the meridian in which the cylinder has no power; that is, 180°. Therefore, the sph / cyl equivalent is   +1.25 DS / +2.00 DC x 180.

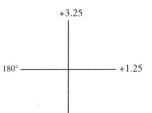

Fig. 3.9

(b) The power diagram is shown in figure 3.10 .

Again, the numerically lower powered meridian is taken to be the sphere; that is, − 0.75 D. The power of the cylinder is

$$C = (S + C) - S$$
$$= (-1.25) - (-0.75) = -0.50 \text{ D.}$$

The cylinder axis meridian is the meridian containing the sphere power only; that is, 150°.
Therefore, the sph / cyl equivalent is   − 0.75 DS / − 0.50 DC x 150.

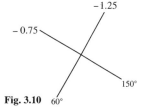

Fig. 3.10

(c) The power diagram is shown in figure 3.11 .
The power of the sphere *S* is taken to be −1.00 D.
The cylinder power is therefore

$$C = (S + C) - S$$
$$= (+1.50) - (-1.00) = +2.50 \text{ D.}$$

The axis is the meridian containing the sphere power only; that is, 45°. Therefore the sph / cyl equivalent is
$$-1.00 \text{ DS} / +2.50 \text{ DC x 45 .}$$

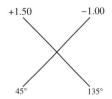

Fig. 3.11

6 The following thin lenses are placed in contact:

(a)   +5.50 DS / +2.00 DC x 115   (b)   −3.50 DS /−0.50 DC x 175
(c)   +0.50 DS /+0.50 DC x 135   (d)   +4.00 DS / −0.50 DC x 85
(e)   −7.50 DS / +1.50 DC x 25   (f)   plano / +0.50 DC x 45 .

What is the resultant power of the combination?

In questions involving thin lenses in contact, the total power is simply the sum of the individual lens powers. With thin sph / cyls, the lenses can only be added together without difficulty when the principal meridians are common; that is, along the same direction. A combination of lenses like the ones given here must be split up so as to group together those lenses with common principal meridians. In this case, the lenses with common principal meridians are respectively (a) and (e), (b) and (d), and (c) and (f). If within each group the cyl axes are matched, the powers can be added together.

(N.B. The choice of which lens to transpose to produce matching axes is arbitrary.)

Lens (a)	+ 5.50 DS / + 2.00 DC x 115
Lens (e) transposed	− 6.00 DS / − 1.50 DC x 115
Addition gives	− 0.50 DS / + 0.50 DC x 115
Lens (b)	− 3.50 DS / − 0.50 DC x 175
Lens (d) transposed	+ 3.50 DS / + 0.50 DC x 175
Addition gives	Plano
Lens (c)	+ 0.50 DS / + 0.50 DC x 135
Lens (f) transposed	+ 0.50 DS / − 0.50 DC x 135
Addition gives	+1.00 DS

Since, in this case, the second pair of lenses neutralise each other, and the third pair has resulted in a sphere, the three groups can now be added together:

Resultant of adding lenses (a) and (e)	−0.50 DS / +0.50 DC x 115
Resultant of adding lenses (b) and (d)	plano
Resultant of adding lenses (c) and (f)	+1.00 DS
Total of combination	+ 0.50 DS / + 0.50 DC x 115

---

7   Transpose the thin lens +2.75 DS / −3.50 DC x 30 into toric form with a +7.50 D base.

While it is possible to complete this operation by employing a memorised set of rules, it is also possible, and perhaps desirable, to obtain the result from first principles. All thin lens toric transposition problems involve only one procedure, that of adding positive spherical power to one surface and an equal amount of negative power to the other. The single rule which is helpful (but not essential) to remember is that when transposing onto a given *base* curve, *the cyl in the sph / cyl form should have the same sign as the base curve.*

In this question then, we require the cylinder expressed in plus form; that is

$$-0.75\,DS / +3.50\,DC \times 120\,.$$

We now represent the sphere and cyl as a power diagram in the schematic form of figure 3.12 . The lens must now be 'bent' by adding equal but opposite spherical powers to each surface to make the cylindrical surface become toroidal with a +7.50 D base curve. By inspection, this is achieved by adding +7.50 DS to the cylindrical surface and −7.50 DS to the spherical surface.

Note that the choice of power to add is the same as the power of the base curve when the cyl has the same sign as the base (here +). This is the reason

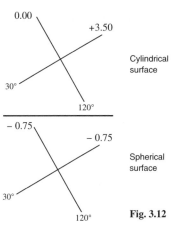

Fig. 3.12

for transposing to that sph/cyl form. The transposition process can be done in a transposition diagram; see figure 3.13 below. Here the left hand power diagrams are the surface powers in the sph/cyl form, the middle part is the transposition term, and the right hand side is the toric form surface powers.

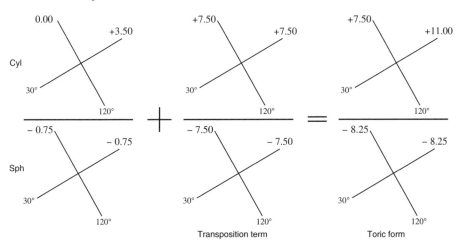

Fig. 3.13   **Diagrammatic representation of thin lens toric transposition.**

The conventional way of writing the specification for this lens is with the toroidal surface expressed as crossed cyls. Furthermore, it is general convention that the front surface is written above the line and the back surface below it, thus:

$$\frac{+7.50\,DC \times 30 \ / +11.00\,DC \times 120}{-8.25\,DS}$$

Using a lens measure, the surface powers would be written as

$$\frac{+7.50\,DC \text{ along } 120° \ / +11.00\,D \text{ along } 30°}{-8.25\,DS}$$

8 Transpose the thin sph/cyl form lens −1.75 DS / +2.50 DC x 60 into toric form with a +9.00 D sphere curve.

When transposing a sph/cyl from onto a given *sphere* curve the procedure is the same as in question 7 except that the amount which is to be added to each surface is found as follows. Inspection of figure 3.14, the schematic representation of the transposition, shows that the required sphere curve (+9.00) in the toric form is the sum of the sphere (−1.75) in the sph/cyl form and the transposition power (+10.75) on this surface. Hence, the transposition power on the sphere surface is found from

transposition power added to sph curve = *sph on toric lens* − *sph in flat lens* .

The procedure can easily be done by inspection, after some practice.

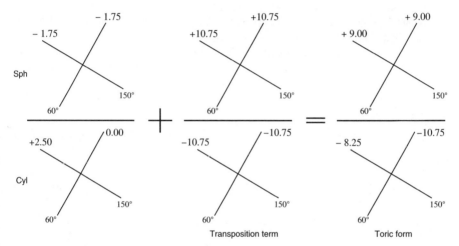

Fig. 3.14 Thin lens toric transposition.

Notice that +10.75 DS is added to the flat sphere power and −10.75 DS added to the cyl surface. The cyl surface becomes toroidal and the lens is a toric.

The written forms of the toric lens are:

$$\frac{+9.00\text{ DS}}{-8.25\text{ DC x }60\,/-10.75\text{ DC x }150} \text{ and } \frac{+9.00\text{ DS}}{-8.25\text{ D along }150°\,/-10.75\text{ DC along }60°} .$$

---

9 Find the principal powers and the sphere/cyl equivalent of the following toric lens.

$$\frac{+6.00\text{ DC x }180\,/+7.75\text{ DC x }90}{-4.50\text{ DS}} .$$

The principal powers may be obtained by drawing power diagrams for each surface in turn and then adding them together. This is simply applying the thin lens equation $F = F_1 + F_2$ to each principal meridian. Figure 3.15 shows the procedure.

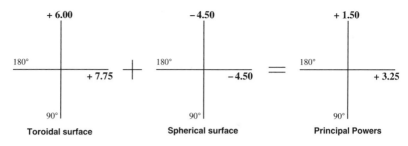

Fig. 3.15

The principal powers are +1.50 D along 90° and +3.25 D along 180°. The sph/cyl equivalent may be obtained from the principal powers by using the method shown in question 3.2 ; that is,   +1.50 DS / +1.75 DC x 90 .

---

10 Transpose the prescription −2.00 DS / +6.00 DC x 180 into toric form with a +5.00 D base curve.

When the power of the base curve is less than the power of the cylinder there are two toric forms possible. One has a conventional convex toroidal surface and the other has a capstan surface. Either form can be obtained using the method set out in question 3.7, but when the capstan form is required it is easier to work from the minus cyl form of the sph/cyl prescription. The conventional form from the prescription as given is:

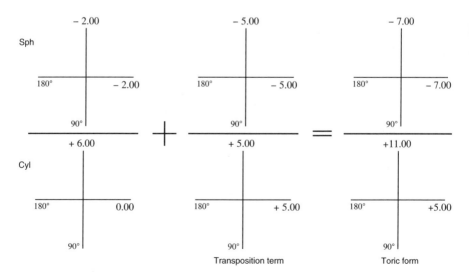

Fig. 3.16   Conventional (barrel or tyre) form with a +5.00 D base.

13

In written form, this is:

$$\frac{+5.00 \text{ DC x } 90 \, / \, + 11.00 \text{ DC x } 180}{-7.00 \text{ DS}} \quad \text{or} \quad \frac{+5.00 \text{ D along } 180° \, / \, + 11.00 \text{ D along } 90°}{-7.00 \text{ DS}} .$$

The capstan form from the transposed prescription, $+4.00$ DS $/ -6.00$ DC x 90, is:

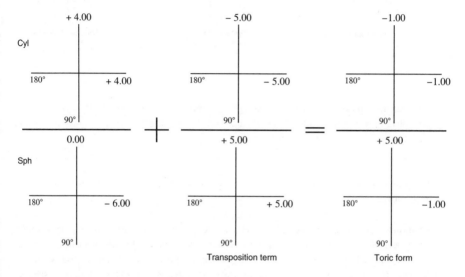

Fig. 3.17   Capstan form with a +5.00 D base.

The written form is:

$$\frac{+5.00 \text{ DC x } 180 \, / \, - 1.00 \text{ DC x } 90}{-1.00 \text{ DS}} \quad \text{or} \quad \frac{+5.00 \text{ D along } 90° \, / \, - 1.00 \text{ D along } 180°}{-1.00 \text{ DS}} .$$

---

11 A thin toric lens is made to the specification:

$$\frac{+6.00 \text{ DC x } 135 \, / \, +7.50 \text{ DC x } 45}{-3.25 \text{ DS}} .$$

When a second thin lens is placed in contact with this lens the power of the combination becomes +1.75 DS / −2.25 DC x 135. What is the power of the second lens?

The principal powers of the first lens are found and subtracted from the principal powers of the combination to obtain the principal powers of the second lens. This follows from the fact that the power of the combination, F, is given by the sum of the two thin lens powers, F_1 and F_2. Hence, $F_2 = F - F_1$.

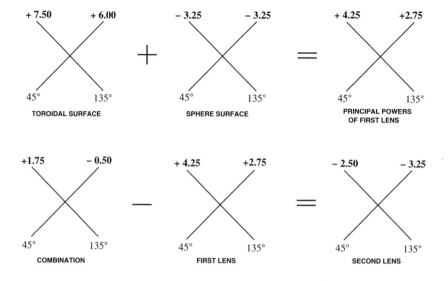

TOROIDAL SURFACE   SPHERE SURFACE   PRINCIPAL POWERS OF FIRST LENS

COMBINATION   FIRST LENS   SECOND LENS

Fig. 3.18   **The upper half of the diagram shows the determination of the principal powers of the first lens, found by adding the surface powers together. The lower half shows subtraction of the first lens power from the power of the combination to find the power of the second lens; that is, $F - F_1 = F_2$.**

Therefore, the power of the second lens is -2.50 DS $/ -0.75$ DC x 135.

---

12   **The resultant power of two plano-cyls placed in contact is plano $/ +3.00$ DC x 90. When one of the cyls is rotated through 90° the resultant power it produces includes a cyl power of -6.00 DC x 90. Find the power of the two plano-cyls, and the spherical power of the resultant.**

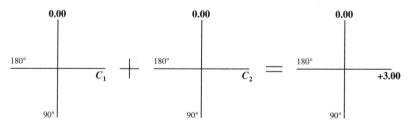

Fig. 3.19   **Addition of two plano-cyls with their axes parallel.**

In figure 3.19, the result of adding the plano-cyls, C_1 and C_2, is

$$C_1 + C_2 = +3.00 \qquad (1).$$

In figure 3.20, we rotate the second plano-cyl through 90° and add them again.

15

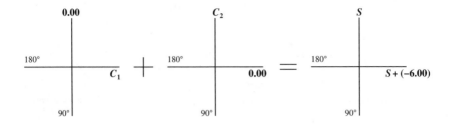

Fig. 3.20 Addition of two plano-cyls with their axes perpendicular. See the calculation below.

S is the spherical power of the resultant. By adding powers on like meridians we have:

$$C_1 = S + (-6.00) = S - 6.00 \qquad (2)$$

$$\text{and} \quad C_2 = S \qquad (3).$$

Substituting for S from equation (3) into equation (2) gives,

$$C_1 = C_2 - 6.00 \qquad (4)$$

and substituting this value for C_1 from equation (4) into equation (1), we have

$$C_2 - 6.00 + C_2 = +3.00, \quad \text{or} \quad 2C_2 = +9.00 .$$

Hence, $\quad C_2 = +4.50 \qquad (5).$

Thus, using equations (5) and (1), we have

$$C_1 = (+3.00) - C_2 = (+3.00) - (+4.50) = -1.50 \text{ D}.$$

From equation (3), the spherical power of the resultant is $S = C_2 = +4.50$ D, and the two cylinder powers have been found to be $+4.50$ D and -1.50 D.

Once having understood the principles, the following quick thin lens toric transposition will be found appealing.

13 **Transpose the lens +2.00 DS / +1.00 DC x 90 into the following toric forms:**
   (a) **+8.00 D sphere curve**   (b) **+7.00 D base curve**
   (c) **−4.00 D sphere curve**   (d) **−3.00 D base curve.**

The starting point is this:
   If the toric form is to have a plus toroidal surface (+ base curve or − sphere curve), then write the sph/cyl form with a plus cyl.
   For a minus toroidal surface form write the sph/cyl form with a minus cyl.

(a) The lens is to have a +8.00 D sphere curve, so the base curve will be negative. Therefore, we write the sph/cyl form with a negative cyl: +3.00 DS / −1.00 DC x 180 .

16

We now write the sph/cyl down like this:

$$\frac{+3.00 \text{ DS}}{/ - 1.00 \text{ DC} \times 180}\ \cdot$$

Next, we invent the mathematical entity, a zero powered plano-cyl with its axis perpendicular to the -1.00 DC 's axis at 180; that is, 0.00 DC x 90 . This lens is written below, thus:

$$\frac{+3.00 \text{ DS}}{0.00 \text{ DC} \times 90\ /\ - 1.00 \text{ DC} \times 180}\ \cdot$$

By inspection, we need to add +5 D to the sphere curve to make it become +8.00 . We must therefore add –5 D to the surface expressed as crossed cyls in order not to change the lens power. We then have the toroidal form:

$$\frac{+8.00 \text{ DS}}{- 5.00 \text{ DC} \times 90\ /\ - 6.00 \text{ DC} \times 180}\ \cdot$$

(b) For a plus base we want a plus cyl transposition; +2.00 DS / +1.00 DC x 90 . Proceeding now with little explanation:

$$\frac{+2.00 \text{ DS}}{/ + 1.00 \text{ DC} \times 90}\ \cdot$$

Then, inserting the zero power plano-cyl:

$$\frac{+2.00 \text{ DS}}{0.00 \text{ DC} \times 180\ /\ + 1.00 \text{ DC} \times 90}\ \cdot$$

We require a +7.00 D base, so we add +7 D to the crossed cyl surface and –7 D to the sphere curve, which gives:

$$\frac{-5.00 \text{ DS}}{+ 7.00 \text{ DC} \times 180\ /\ + 8.00 \text{ DC} \times 90}\ \cdot$$

Writing this the conventional way around, we have:

$$\frac{+7.00 \text{ DC} \times 180\ /\ + 8.00 \text{ DC} \times 90}{- 5.00 \text{ DS}}\ \cdot$$

(c) This requires a – 4.00 D sphere curve, which means it will have a plus base toroidal surface, so we start with the lens in plus cyl form:

$$\frac{+2.00 \text{ DS}}{/ + 1.00 \text{ DC} \times 90}\ \cdot$$

Then, inserting the zero powered cyl:

$$\frac{+2.00 \text{ DS}}{0.00 \text{ DC} \times 180\ /\ + 1.00 \text{ DC} \times 90}\ \cdot$$

Now, by inspection, we add –6 D to the sphere curve to produce the required – 4.00 D sphere curve, and then we add + 6 D to the other surface:

$$\frac{- 4.00 \text{ DS}}{+ 6.00 \text{ DC} \times 180\ /\ + 7.00 \text{ DC} \times 90}\ \cdot$$

We then write this the conventional way around:

$$\frac{+6.00 \text{ DC x } 180 \text{ / } + 7.00 \text{ DC x } 90}{- 4.00 \text{ DS}} \cdot$$

(d) This requires a −3.00 D base, so without explanation, to show how little work is involved, we have:

$$\frac{+3.00 \text{ DS}}{0.00 \text{ DC x } 90 \text{ / } - 1.00 \text{ DC x } 180} \cdot$$

$$\frac{+6.00 \text{ DS}}{- 3.00 \text{ DC x } 90 \text{ / } - 4.00 \text{ DC x } 180} \cdot$$

---

14 **Using the *Easy Toric Transposition Method* of question 13 above**
 (i) **transpose the lens −5.00 DS / −2.25 DC x 180 into toric form on a +3.00 D sphere curve**
 (ii) **then transpose this toric form into a new toric form on a −10.00 D base curve.**

(i) Since the first form will result in a minus toroidal surface, the minus cyl transposition is already correct for the *Easy Method*. Hence,

write the zero powered crossed cyl form $\quad \dfrac{-5.00 \text{ DS}}{0.00 \text{ DC x } 90 \text{ / } - 2.25 \text{ DC x } 180} \cdot$

Deduce how much plus power needs to be added to −5.00 to make it come out as +3.00: the amount is +8.00, so

$$\frac{\text{Add} + 8.00}{\text{Add} - 8.00} \quad \Rightarrow \quad \frac{+3.00 \text{ DS}}{-8.00 \text{ DC x } 90 \text{ / } - 10.25 \text{ DC x } 180} \cdot$$

We see that +8.00 has been added to the sphere surface and −8.00 to the crossed-cyl surface. That's part (i) completed!

(ii) The above lens has a −8.00 D toroidal base curve. Adding −2.00 to this will make it −10.00, so we proceed as shown below:

$$\frac{\text{Add} + 2.00}{\text{Add} - 2.00} \quad \text{to} \quad \frac{+3.00 \text{ DS}}{-8.00 \text{ DC x } 90 \text{ / } - 10.25 \text{ DC x } 180}$$

$$\Rightarrow \quad \frac{+5.00 \text{ DS}}{-10.00 \text{ DC x } 90 \text{ / } - 12.25 \text{ DC x } 180} \cdot$$

Of course, we are adding a plus spherical power to one surface and an equal amount of minus spherical power to the other surface, just as we did with the *transposition term* in earlier questions in this section. Just what we add is determined by inspection of either the toroidal base curve or the sphere curve required. Thin lens toric transposition can be summarised in symbols as follows: $\quad F = F_1 + F_2 = (F_1 + \delta F) + (F_2 - \delta F)$, where adding and subtracting δF transposes the lens into another form of the same power F.

N.B. In questions 1 to 16 we do not apply a sign convention with either the approximate or accurate sag formulae, so the surface power F should only have its magnitude entered. This can be made explicit by writing the approximate sag equation in the form

$$s = \frac{y^2 |F|}{2000\,(n - 1)}.$$

Conversely, questions 17 and 18 show the use of the sign convention with the approximate sag formula.

1   A lens measure calibrated for refractive index 1.523 reads +4.50 D when placed on the surface of a lens made of glass of refractive index 1.654 . What is the actual surface power?

Since a lens measure measures the sag of a surface and is calibrated to be read in dioptres of power for a specific refractive index, it is possible to find the radius of curvature of a surface. In this case

$$r = \frac{n'-n}{F} = \frac{1.523 - 1}{+4.5} = +0.1162 \text{ m.}$$

The true power of this surface will be found by relating this radius of curvature to the refractive index of the glass from which the lens is made:

Thus $F = \dfrac{n'-n}{r} = \dfrac{1.523 - 1}{+0.1162} = +5.63 \text{ D.}$

---

2   A lens measure gives a maximum reading of +6.25 D when it is applied to the outside of a plastic tube 16.75 cm in diameter. For what refractive index is the lens measure calibrated?

If the diameter of the tube is 16.75 cm, its radius is 8.375 cm or 0.08375 m. Relating this radius of curvature to the power which was indicated on the instrument will give the refractive index for which it is calibrated.

From $F = \dfrac{n'-n}{r} = \dfrac{n_g - 1}{r}$, we have $n_g = rF + 1 = (0.08375 \times 6.25) + 1 = 1.523$.

---

3   A lens measure is placed on the outside of a metal tube and a maximum reading of +9.00 D is obtained. If the instrument is calibrated for glass of refractive index 1.523, what is the diameter of the metal tube?

The relationship between radius of curvature, refractive index, and power is given by

$$F = \frac{n' - n}{r} = \frac{n_g - 1}{r} \ , \quad \text{where } n_g \text{ is the refractive index of the glass.}$$

Therefore, $r = \dfrac{n_g - 1}{F} = \dfrac{1.523 - 1}{+9.00} = +0.0581 \text{ m} = +5.81 \text{ cm}$

and the tube diameter is twice this; that is, $2 \times 5.81 = 11.62$ cm.

---

4   A lens measure calibrated for refractive index 1.523 has a distance of 20 mm between its fixed legs. After the instrument is accidentally dropped, the separation of the legs is 21 mm. What power will now be recorded by the instrument when it is placed on the +6.00 D surface of an ophthalmic crown lens?

By using the approximate sag formula, first, find the sag which this instrument records after it has been dropped :

$$s = \frac{y^2 \, |F|}{2000 \, (n - 1)} = \frac{(10.5)^2 \times 6}{2000 \times (1.523 - 1)} = 0.632 \text{ mm, where } y = 21/2 = 10.5 \text{ mm.}$$

Now, using this sag and the value of $y = 10$ mm for which the instrument is calibrated, the power reading will be

$$|F| = \frac{2000 \, (n - 1) \, s}{y^2} = \frac{2000 \times (1.523 - 1) \times 0.632}{10^2} = 6.61 \text{ D.}$$

The power is plus since the surface is convex.

---

5   The fixed legs of a lens measure are separated by 20 mm. It is calibrated for refractive index 1.523 . When placed on the curved surface of a plano-convex lens, the central leg is depressed 0.5 mm from its position on a plane surface. The power of the lens is found by neutralisation to be +5.75 D. What is the refractive index of the glass from which the lens is made?

N.B. The neutralising power, or front vertex power, of a lens is the same as the front surface power, F_1 , when the lens is plano-convex; that is, when $F_2 = 0$. Strictly, we should call this a convexo-plane lens!

The given refractive index for which the instrument is calibrated is not required since we are told the sag of the surface; that is, $s = 0.5$ mm. Firstly, find the radius of curvature of the surface by using the approximate sag relationship:

$$r = \frac{y^2}{2s} = \frac{10^2}{2 \times 0.5} = 100 \text{ mm } = 0.100 \text{ m.}$$

Now, find the refractive index from the surface power relationship:

$$F = \frac{n' - n}{r} = \frac{n_g - 1}{r} , \text{ so we have } n_g = rF + 1 = (0.100 \times 5.75) + 1 = 1.575 .$$

Alternative method
It can be done in one step using the approximate sag formula in the form

$$s = \frac{y^2 |F|}{2000 (n_g - 1)}$$

which rearranges to give $n_g = 1 + \dfrac{y^2 |F|}{2000\, s} = 1 + \dfrac{10^2 \times 5.75}{2000 \times 0.5} = 1.575 .$

---

6   In a practical case, the Back Vertex Power of a lens is found to be −8.00 using a focimeter. Using a lens measure the sum of the surface powers is −7.50. What is the refractive index of the lens material.

Using F_{TRUE} for the value obtained with the focimeter, and F_{LM} for the value obtained

with the lens measure, we rearrange the equation $F_{\text{TRUE}} = \left(\dfrac{n_{\text{TRUE}} - 1}{1.523 - 1} \right) F_{\text{LM}}$

$$\Rightarrow n_{\text{TRUE}} = 1 + 0.523 \times \frac{F_{\text{TRUE}}}{F_{\text{LM}}} = 1 + 0.523 \times \frac{(-8.00)}{(-7.50)} = 1.56 .$$

---

7   Find the centre thickness of a +7.50 D plano-convex spherical lens for which the refractive index is 1.523 . Its edge thickness is 0.7 mm and the lens size is 42 mm round. Use the approximate sag formula. (Note: the expression "42 mm round" is taken to indicate that the lens is cut round in shape and 42 mm in diameter.)

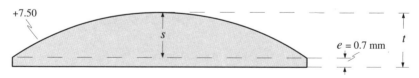

Fig. 4.1   Major section through the plano-convex lens in question 7.

From the diagram, it can be seen that $t = e + s$. Using the approximate sag formula,

we have $s = \dfrac{y^2 |F|}{2000 (n_g - 1)} \quad \dfrac{21^2 \times 7.50}{2000 \times (1.523 - 1)} = 3.16$ mm, where $y = \dfrac{42}{2} = 21$.

Hence, the centre thickness is $t = e + s = 0.7 + 3.16 = 3.86$ mm.

8 A meniscus lens has surface powers +6.00 D and −10.00 D. Its centre thickness is 0.8 mm and it is flat edged 44 mm round. Find *accurately* its edge thickness and the thickness of the thinnest flate plate of glass from which it can be ground. $n_g = 1.523$.

We shall call the thinnest flat plate of glass from which the lens can be obtained the Minimum Plate Thickness (MPT).

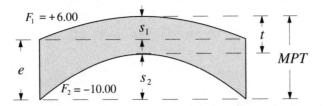

Fig. 4.2   Diagram used in question 8.   Note the diagram is not to scale. 'Thickening up' the lens makes the dimensions easier to sort out.

From figure 4.2, the following relationships are evident:

$$MPT = s_2 + t, \quad \text{or} \quad MPT = s_1 + e, \quad \text{so that} \quad e = MPT - s_1 .$$

To find s_1 and s_2 by the accurate sag formula it is first necessary to calculate the radii of curvature of the front and back surfaces:

$$r_1 = \frac{n_1' - n_1}{F_1} = \frac{1.523 - 1}{+6} = +0.0872 \text{ m} = +87.2 \text{ mm}$$

$$\text{and} \quad r_2 = \frac{n_2' - n_2}{F_2} = \frac{1 - 1.523}{-10} = +0.0523 \text{ m} = +52.3 \text{ mm}$$

Then, using the accurate sag formula,

$$s_1 = r_1 - \sqrt{r_1^2 - y^2} = 87.2 - \sqrt{87.2^2 - 22^2} = 87.2 - 84.4 = 2.8 \text{ mm}.$$

$$\text{and} \quad s_2 = r_2 - \sqrt{r_2^2 - y^2} = 52.3 - \sqrt{52.3^2 - 22^2} = 52.3 - 47.4 = 4.9 \text{ mm}.$$

Therefore, $MPT = s_2 + t = 4.9 + 0.8 = 5.7$ mm

and $e = MPT - s_1 = 5.7 - 2.8 = 2.9$ mm.

9 **A flat sph/cyl +7.00 DS / −4.00 DC x 90 is made up as a 42 mm round lens with a thin edge substance of 1.8 mm in glass of refractive index 1.523. Calculate the centre thickness and the thick edge substance.**

A flat sph/cyl has its spherical power worked on one surface and its cylindrical power on the other. Therefore, diagrams are required illustrating sections though each of the principal meridians of the lens. In this way, the relationships between the thick and thin edge substances and the two sags may be deduced by inspection of figures 4.3 and 4.4.

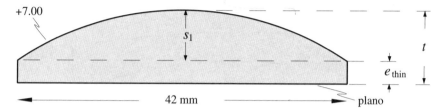

Fig. 4.3 Section through the lens along the 90° principal meridian.

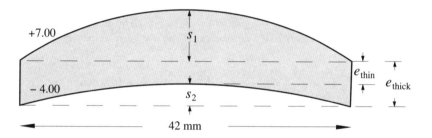

Fig. 4.4 Section through the lens along the 180° principal meridian.

From figure 4.3, the centre thickness of the lens is

$$t = s_1 + e_{thin} = \frac{y^2 |F|}{2000(n_g - 1)} + e_{thin} = \frac{21^2 \times 7}{2000 \times (1.523 - 1)} + 1.8 = 4.75 \text{ mm.}$$

By inspection of figure 4.4, the thick edge substance is given by $e_{thick} = e_{thin} + s_2$.

So we need the sag (s_2) of the back surface :

$$s_2 = \frac{y^2 |F_2|}{2000(n_g - 1)} = \frac{21^2 \times 4}{2000(1.523 - 1)} = 1.7 \text{ mm.}$$

Hence, the thick edge substance is $e_{thick} = e_{thin} + s_2 = 1.8 + 1.7 = 3.5$ mm.

23

10 The lens **+2.50 DS / – 4.00 DC x 180** is made up as a flat sph/cyl. It is edged **46 mm × 40 mm oval, and the edge thickness at each end of its vertical principal meridian is 4 mm.** $n_g = 1.523$, **and the optical centre is at the geometrical centre of the lens. Find the edge thickness at the extremities of its horizontal principal meridian.**

As before, any problem concerned with sag and thickness can be dealt with more easily if diagrams are made of the lens sectioned though each of its principal meridians; see figures 4.5 and 4.6 .

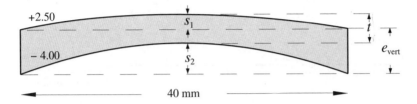

Fig. 4.5 Section through the lens along the vertical principal meridian.

Since this diagram, and figure 4.6, represent sections through the principal meridians of the same lens, the centre thickness t is common. Using the approximate sag formula, from figure 4.5,

$$s_1 = \frac{y^2 |F_1|}{2000 (n_g - 1)} = \frac{20^2 \times 2.5}{2000 (1.523 - 1)} = 0.96 \text{ mm.}$$

$$s_2 = \frac{y^2 |F_2|}{2000 (n_g - 1)} = \frac{20^2 \times 4}{2000 (1.523 - 1)} = 1.53 \text{ mm.}$$

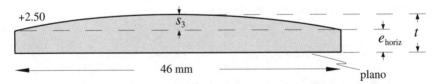

Fig. 4.6 Section through the lens along the horizontal principal meridian.

$$s_3 = \frac{y^2 |F_3|}{2000 (n_g - 1)} = \frac{23^2 \times 2.5}{2000 (1.523 - 1)} = 1.26 \text{ mm.}$$

Note that s_1 and s_2 are the sags of the front and back surfaces in the vertical meridian of this lens and it is necessary to calculate them using the vertical lens half-diameter, $y = 20$ mm. s_3 is the sag of the front surface in the horizontal meridian, and consequently it is calculated

24

using the horizontal lens half-diameter, $y = 23$ mm. Subscripts 1, 2, and 3 are applied to the corresponding powers, F, in these meridians. Thus, F_1 is the power of the front surface in the vertical meridian, F_3 is the power of the front surface in the horizontal meridian, and F_2 is the back surface power in the vertical meridian.

From figure 4.5, it can be deduced that $t = s_1 + (e_{vert} - s_2) = 0.964 + (4 - 1.53) = 3.43$ mm, and from figure 4.6, $e_{horiz} = t - s_3 = 3.43 - 1.26 = 2.17$ mm.

---

11 **The flat sph/cyl −6.25 DS / +1.50 DC x 180 has a finished lens size of 46 mm × 40 mm oval. It has been decentred 4 mm in and its centre thickness is 0.8 mm. Calculate its edge thickness at both ends of the Horizontal Centre Line (datum line). The refractive index is 1.523.**

Note (i) that the cylinder does not contribute to the edge thickness in the horizontal meridian when its axis is 180° and (ii) the optical centre is on the horizontal centre line. The notation is shown in figure 4.7. Thus, using the approximate sag formula,

$$s_1 = \frac{y^2 |F_1|}{2000\,(n_g - 1)} = \frac{19^2 \times 6.25}{2000\,(1.523 - 1)} = 2.16 \text{ mm}$$

$$s_2 = \frac{y^2 |F_2|}{2000\,(n_g - 1)} = \frac{27^2 \times 6.25}{2000\,(1.523 - 1)} = 4.36 \text{ mm}.$$

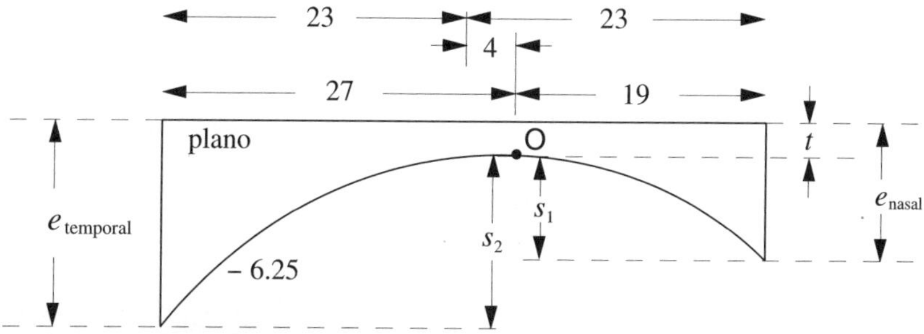

Fig. 4.7 **Horizontal section through the lens along the Horizontal Centre Line.**

From figure 4.7, $e_{nasal} = t + s_1 = 0.8 + 2.16 = 2.96$ mm,

and $e_{temporal} = t + s_2 = 0.8 + 4.36 = 5.16$ mm.

---

12 A flat sph/cyl lens +5.00 DS / +3.00 DC x 120, made of glass of refractive index 1.523, has a datum lens size 48 mm × 40 mm. Its optical centre is 2 mm above datum line (Horizontal Centre Line) and its edge thickness at the lower edge of the vertical meridian is 2 mm. What is the thickness at its optical centre?

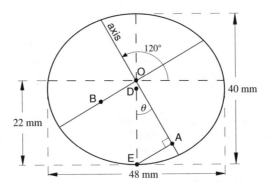

Fig. 4.8

In figure 4.8, O is the optical centre and E is the point at which the edge thickness is known. EA has been constructed perpendicular to the cylinder axis, and OB = EA.

Since the power of the cylinder lies along its power meridian or any meridian parallel to it, the sag of the cylindrical surface at the point E is the same as if the point in question were at B. EA can be found from the geometry of the figure:

Since $OE = OD + DE = 2 + 20 = 22$ mm, $EA = OE \sin \theta = 22 \sin 30° = 11$ mm.

A section through this lens along the 30° meridian would show that it is biconvex and the centre thickness, t, of a biconvex lens is obtained by adding the two sags to a known edge thickness, e. The sag, s_1, of the spherical surface is given by

$$s_1 = \frac{y^2 |F_1|}{2000 (n_g - 1)} = \frac{22^2 \times 5}{2000 (1.523 - 1)} = 2.31 \text{ mm, where } y = OE = 22 \text{ mm.}$$

The sag, s_2, of the cylindrical surface is given by

$$s_2 = \frac{y^2 |F_2|}{2000 (n_g - 1)} = \frac{11^2 \times 3}{2000 (1.523 - 1)} = 0.35 \text{ mm, where } y = OB = 11 \text{mm.}$$

Hence, $t = e + s_1 + s_2 = 2 + 2.31 + 0.35 = 4.66$ mm.

13 The prescription +2.25 DS / +3.50 DC x 45 is made up in toric form with a +6.00 D base curve. It is to be made in glass of refractive index 1.523 and edged 44 mm round. Its thin edge substance is 1.5 mm. Calculate its thick edge substance. What is the thinnest parallel sided plate from which it could be ground?

The surface powers must be found first. The method was shown in question 3.7: thus, the toric form is

$$\frac{+6.00\ DC \times 135\ /\ +9.50\ DC \times 45}{-3.75\ DS} \quad \text{or} \quad \frac{+6.00\ D\ \text{along}\ 45°\ /\ +9.50\ D\ \text{along}\ 135°}{-3.75\ DS}.$$

A diagram of sections through each of the principal meridians should now be made. In the case of a toric lens it may be helpful if one section is superimposed on the other; see figure 4.9.

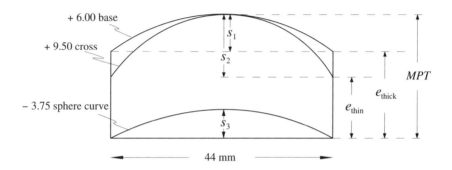

Fig. 4.9 The two principal sections of a toric lens superimposed.

From the figure, $MPT = e_{thin} + s_2$ (1) and $e_{thick} = MPT - s_1$ (2).

Therefore, we see that the sag s_3 plays no part in this calculation.

$$\text{Now,} \quad s_1 = \frac{y^2\ |F_{base}|}{2000\ (n_g - 1)} = \frac{22^2 \times 6}{2000\ (1.523 - 1)} = 2.8\ \text{mm}$$

$$\text{and} \quad s_2 = \frac{y^2\ |F_{cross}|}{2000\ (n_g - 1)} = \frac{22^2 \times 9.5}{2000\ (1.523 - 1)} = 4.4\ \text{mm}.$$

Hence, using equation (1), we have

the Minimum Plate Thickness, $MPT = e_{thin} + s_2 = 1.5 + 4.4 = 5.9$ mm.

From equation (2), the thick edge substance is $e_{thick} = MPT - s_1 = 5.9 - 2.8 = 3.1$ mm.

14 A toric lens of power **−5.75 DS / +4.00 DC x 180** is made with a **−6.00 D base curve**. It is to be made in plastics material of refractive index 1.56. The boxed lens size is **46 × 38 oval** and the lens is not decentred. If the minimum edge thickness is 2 mm, calculate the centre thickness and the edge thickness in the other principal meridian using the accurate sag formula.

Find the surface powers using the method in question 3.7 . This gives

$$\frac{+4.25\,\text{DS}}{-6.00\,\text{DC x 180} / -10.00\,\text{DC x 90}} \quad \text{or} \quad \frac{+4.25\,\text{DS}}{-6.00\,\text{D along 90} / -10.00\,\text{D along 180}}$$

The composite diagram of the lens sectioned along each of its principal meridians is as follows:

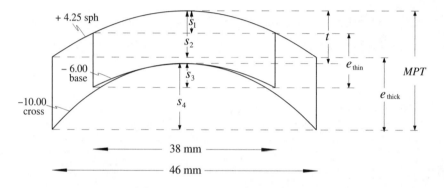

Fig. 4.10   Sections through the two principal meridians of the toric lens.

Although the diagram becomes more complicated when the lens is not circular, once it has been obtained the following relationships will be seen to apply to this lens:

$$t = s_1 + (e_{\text{thin}} - s_3) \qquad MPT = t + s_4 \qquad e_{\text{thick}} = MPT - s_2 \,.$$

Find the radii of curvature: we shall use subscripts b, c, and *s* for base, cross, and sphere curve, respectively.

$$r_b = \frac{n_b' - n_b}{F_b} = \frac{1 - 1.56}{-6}\,\text{m} = 93.33\,\text{mm}.$$

$$r_c = \frac{n_c' - n_c}{F_c} = \frac{1 - 1.56}{-10}\,\text{m} = 56.00\,\text{mm}.$$

$$r_s = \frac{n_s' - n_s}{F_s} = \frac{1.56 - 1}{4.25}\,\text{m} = 131.76\,\text{mm}.$$

Find the sags: subscripts v and h stand for vertical and horizontal, respectively.

$$s_1 = r_s - \sqrt{r_s^2 - y_v^2} = 131.76 - \sqrt{131.76^2 - 19^2} = 131.76 - 130.38 = 1.38 \text{ mm}.$$

$$s_2 = r_s - \sqrt{r_s^2 - y_h^2} = 131.76 - \sqrt{131.76^2 - 23^2} = 131.76 - 129.76 = 2.00 \text{ mm}.$$

$$s_3 = r_b - \sqrt{r_b^2 - y_v^2} = 93.33 - \sqrt{93.33^2 - 19^2} = 93.33 - 91.38 = 1.95 \text{ mm}.$$

$$s_4 = r_c - \sqrt{r_c^2 - y_h^2} = 56.00 - \sqrt{56.00^2 - 23^2} = 56.00 - 51.06 = 4.94 \text{ mm}.$$

Substituting these values in the expressions obtained from figure 4.10, we have

$$t = s_1 + (e_{thin} - s_3) = 1.38 + (2 - 1.95) = 1.43 \text{ mm},$$
$$MPT = t + s_4 = 1.43 + 4.94 = 6.37 \text{ mm},$$
$$\text{and } e_{thick} = MPT - s_2 = 6.37 - 2.00 = 4.37 \text{ mm}.$$

---

15 **A lens has a concave toroidal surface, the base curve of which is –7.50 D. Its other surface is plane. It is edged 44 mm round, has a centre thickness 0.8 mm, and is made of glass of refractive index 1.523 . If its thick edge substance is 6.06 mm, find its thin edge substance and the power of the Rx cylinder. Use the accurate sag formula.**

Find s_b : the subscript b stands for base. See figure 4.11.

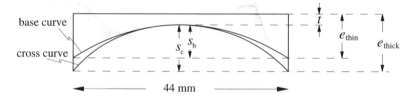

base curve

cross curve

44 mm

Fig. 4.11 **Composite diagram of sections through both principal meridians of the lens.**

We first need to find the radius r_b of the base curve, thus

$$r_b = \frac{n_b' - n_b}{F_b} = \frac{1 - 1.523}{-7.50} \text{ m} = +69.73 \text{ mm}.$$

Using r_b in the accurate sag formula gives the sag s_b of the base curve:

$$s_b = r_b - \sqrt{r_b^2 - y^2} = 69.73 - \sqrt{69.73^2 - 22^2} = 69.73 - 66.17 = 3.56 \text{ mm}.$$

From figure 4.11, $e_{thin} = t + s_b = 0.8 + 3.56 = 4.36 \text{ mm}.$

To obtain the cylinder power it is first necessary to find the power of the cross curve. In figure 4.11, the sag of the cross curve is s_c and $s_c = e_{thick} - t = 6.06 - 0.8 = 5.26 \text{ mm}.$

Using the subscript c for cross curve, find the power of the cross curve:

$$r_c = \frac{y^2 + s_c^2}{2\,s_c} = \frac{22^2 + 5.26^2}{2 \times 5.26} = 48.64 \text{ mm}$$

so $\qquad F_c = \dfrac{n_c' - n_c}{r_c} = \dfrac{1 - 1.523}{+0.0464} = -10.75 \text{ D.}$

The cylinder power is the difference between the cross curve and the base curve powers; that is $-10.75 - (-7.50) = -3.25$ D.

---

16 A plano-convex lens, figure 4.12, has $BVP = +10.00$ D, edge thickness 3 mm when flat-edged 50 mm round, and is made of glass of refractive index 1.5 . Find the centre thickness (t) and the front surface power (F_1) . Use may be made of the approximate sag formula.

We know that:

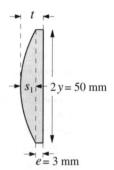

(i) $\quad F_1 = \dfrac{F_v' - F_2}{1 + \dfrac{t/1000}{n_g}\,(F_v' - F_2)} = \dfrac{10 - 0}{1 + \dfrac{t/1000}{1.5}\,(10 - 0)}$

$= \dfrac{10}{1 + \dfrac{6.667}{1000}\,t} = \dfrac{10\,000}{1000 + 6.667\,t}$ with t in mm,

and

(ii) $\quad F_1 = \dfrac{2000\,(n_g - 1)\,s_1}{y^2} = \dfrac{2000\,(1.5 - 1)(t - 3)}{25^2}$

Fig. 4.12

$= \dfrac{1000\,(t - 3)}{625} = 1.6t - 4.8$ (having used $s_1 = t - e = t - 3$ mm).

Since the left hand sides of equations (i) and (ii) are equal, we can equate the right hand sides: thus

$$\frac{10\,000}{1000 + 6.667\,t} = 1.6t - 4.8 .$$

Multiplying both sides by $(1000 + 6.667\,t)$ gives

$$10\,000 = (1.6t - 4.8)\,(1000 + 6.667\,t)$$

$$= 1600t - 4800 + 10.667\,t^2 - 32t$$

Rearranging the terms,

$$10.667\,t^2 + 1568\,t - 14800 = 0 \qquad\qquad \text{(iii).}$$

Now, the general quadratic equation $ax^2 + bx + c = 0$ has the solutions

$$x = \frac{-b \pm \sqrt{b^2 - 4ac}}{2a} .$$

Putting $a = 10.667$, $b = 1568$, $c = -14800$, the solution of equation (iii) is

$$t = \frac{-1568 \pm \sqrt{1568^2 - (4 \times 10.667 \times (-14800))}}{2 \times 10.667}$$

$$= \frac{-1568 \pm 1757.9}{2 \times 10.667}$$

$$= 8.90 \text{ mm, having used the positive root.}$$

Putting $t = 8.90$ mm in equation (ii) gives

$$F_1 = 1.6\,t - 4.8 = (1.6 \times 8.90) - 4.8 = +9.44 \text{ D.}$$

---

17 If a sign convention is applied to sags, the sag taking the same sign as the radius of curvature of the surface, then the centre thickness (t), the edge thickness (e), and the front and back surface sags (s_1 and s_2) are related by the equation $t = e + s_1 - s_2$. This equation holds for all lens forms, the front surface being drawn on the left. Use this equation, and the approximate sag formula

$$s = \frac{y^2 F}{2000\,(n' - n)} \quad \textit{(note that the surface power F now takes a sign)}$$

to find the centre thickness of a biconvex lens, flat-edged 50 mm round, made in glass of refractive index 1.5, with an edge thickness 1 mm, and surface powers $F_1 = +3.00$ DS and $F_2 = +2.00$ DS.

Calculate the sags, imagining the lens as in figure 4.13; that is, as though light were coming from the left so that the sign convention applies.

$$s_1 = \frac{y^2 F_1}{2000\,(n_1' - n_1)} = \frac{25^2 \times (+3)}{2000\,(1.5 - 1)} = +1.88 \text{ mm}$$

and

$$s_2 = \frac{y^2 F_2}{2000\,(n_2' - n_2)} = \frac{25^2 \times (+2)}{2000\,(1 - 1.5)} = -1.25 \text{ mm}$$

Since $e = 1$ mm, we have

$$t = e + s_1 - s_2 = 1 + (+1.88) - (-1.25) = 4.13 \text{ mm.}$$

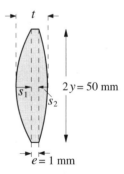

Fig. 4.13

18(i) Apply the sign convention for sags used in question 17 to find the edge thickness in the principal meridians of the lens where the front surface is +3.00 DS and the back surface is –6.00 D along 180° / –9.00 D along 90°. The centre thickness is 1.5 mm, the refractive index is 1.523, and the lens is flat-edged 54 mm round. Use the approximate sag formula.

(ii) Work the problem again where the refractive index is 1.7 instead of 1.523.

(i) <u>Horizontal meridian</u>

$$s_1 = \frac{y^2 F_1}{2000\,(n_1' - n_1)} = \frac{27^2 \times (+3)}{2000\,(1.523 - 1)} = +2.09 \text{ mm}$$

$$\text{and} \quad s_2 = \frac{y^2 F_2}{2000\,(n_2' - n_2)} = \frac{25^2 \times (-6)}{2000\,(1 - 1.523)} = +4.18 \text{ mm}.$$

Note that since these equations are linear, we could have found s_2 from

$$\frac{s_2}{s_1} = \frac{\dfrac{y^2 F_1}{2000\,(n_1' - n_1)}}{\dfrac{y^2 F_2}{2000\,(n_2' - n_2)}} = -\frac{F_1}{F_2} \quad \text{since } (n_2' - n_2) = -(n_1' - n_1) \text{ for a lens in air.}$$

That is, $\quad s_2 = -\dfrac{F_2}{F_1}\,s_1 = -\left(\dfrac{-6}{+3}\right) \times (+2.09) = +4.18 \text{ mm}.$

Thus, $\quad e = t - s_1 + s_2 = 1.5 - (+2.09) + (+4.18) = 3.59 \text{ mm}.$

Note that e and t do not take signs.

<u>Vertical meridian</u>

s_1 is again +2.09 mm, since the front surface is spherical and the diameter is still $2y = 54$ mm. The sag of the back surface in the vertical meridian is

$$s_2 = -\frac{F_2}{F_1}\,s_1 = -\left(\frac{-9}{+3}\right) \times (+2.09) = +6.27 \text{ mm}.$$

Hence, $\quad e = t - s_1 + s_2 = 1.5 - (+2.09) + (+6.27) = 5.68 \text{ mm}.$

(ii) When the refractive index is 1.7:

<u>Horizontal meridian</u>

$$s_1 = \frac{y^2 F_1}{2000\,(n_1' - n_1)} = \frac{27^2 \times (+3)}{2000\,(1.7 - 1)} = +1.56 \text{ mm}$$

$$s_2 = -\frac{F_2}{F_1}\,s_1 = -\left(\frac{-6}{+3}\right) \times (+1.56) = +3.12 \text{ mm}.$$

Thus, $\quad e = t - s_1 + s_2 = 1.5 - (+1.56) + (+3.12) = 3.06 \text{ mm}.$

Vertical meridian

s_1 is the same again, that is $+1.56$ mm.

Then $\quad s_2 \;=\; -\dfrac{F_2}{F_1}\, s_1 \;=\; -\left(\dfrac{-9}{+3}\right) \times (+1.56) \;=\; +4.68$ mm.

Hence, $\quad e = t - s_1 + s_2 = 1.5 - (+1.56) + (+4.68) = 4.62$ mm.

---

19 **A $+6.00$ DS lens is made in three forms, each with $\varnothing 60$ mm, $e = 1$ mm, and $n_p = 1.6$:**

(a) **Spheric, with back surface power $F_2 = -4.75$ DS, and front surface power $F_1 = +10.35$ DS .**

(b) **Conicoid with $F_2 = -2.50$ DS, $F_{1,0} = +8.26$ D (at the vertex), and asphericity $p = 0.240$.**

(c) **Deformed conicoid with $F_2 = -2.50$ DS, $F_{1,0} = +8.30$ (at the vertex), and asphericity $p = 0.240$. The polynomial surface parameters are:**
$$B = 2.0 \times 10^{-9}, \; C = 8.0 \times 10^{-11}, D = 4.0 \times 10^{-13}, \text{ and } E = -2.0 \times 10^{-15}.$$

Calculate the centre thickness of each lens.

(a) The spheric is straightforward: the centre thickness is $t = s_1 + e - s_2$.
To accurately calculate the sags we need the surface radii :
$$r_1 \;=\; \frac{n_1' - n_1}{F_1} \;=\; \frac{1.6 - 1.0}{+10.35} \;=\; +0.05797 \text{ m} \;=\; +57.97 \text{ mm.}$$

and $\quad r_2 \;=\; \dfrac{n_2' - n_2}{F_2} \;=\; \dfrac{1.0 - 1.6}{-4.75} \;=\; +0.12632 \text{ m} \;=\; +126.32 \text{ mm.}$

Then, with the semi-chord diameter $y = 30$ mm,
$$s_1 \;=\; r_1 - \sqrt{r_1^2 - y^2} \;=\; 57.97 - \sqrt{57.97^2 - 30^2} \;=\; 8.37 \text{ mm.}$$

and $\quad s_2 \;=\; r_2 - \sqrt{r_2^2 - y^2} \;=\; 126.32 - \sqrt{126.32^2 - 30^2} \;=\; 3.61 \text{ mm.}$

So, the centre thickness is $t = s_1 + e - s_2 = 8.37 + 1.00 - 3.61 = 5.76$ mm.

(b) The equation for the conicoid front surface, here a prolate ellipse since $0 < p < 1$, is $y^2 = 2 r_0 x - p x^2$ where $y = 30$ mm, x is the sag, r_0 is the front surface radius at the vertex (denoted by $r_{1,0}$ in the calculation below), and $p = 0.240$ is the asphericity. We first calculate $r_{1,0}$ for the front surface using the relationship between surface power and radius of curvature:
$$r_{1,0} \;=\; \frac{n_1' - n_1}{F_{1,0}} \;=\; \frac{1.6 - 1.0}{+8.26} \;=\; +0.07264 \text{ m} \;=\; +72.64 \text{ mm.}$$

The radius of the spherical back surface is:
$$r_2 \;=\; \frac{n_2' - n_2}{F_2} \;=\; \frac{1.0 - 1.6}{-2.50} \;=\; +0.24000 \text{ m} \;=\; +240.00 \text{ mm.}$$

The equation involving the sag should be rearranged into the form of a general quadratic equation to enable the solution to be easily written: $p x_1^2 - 2 r_{1,0}\, x_1 + y^2 = 0$, using the subscript 1 for the sag x_1, and $r_{1,0}$ for the vertex radius of the front aspherical surface. Writing the solution of a quadratic equation to give the sag x_1: taking the negative root,

$$x_1 = \frac{-(-2r_{1,0}) - \sqrt{(-2r_{1,0})^2 - 4 \times p \times y^2}}{2p}$$

$$x_1 = \frac{-(-2 \times 72.64) - \sqrt{(-2 \times 72.64)^2 - 4 \times 0.240 \times 30^2}}{2 \times 0.240}$$

$$x_1 = \frac{145.28 - 142.28}{0.480} = 6.25 \text{ mm.}$$

The sag s_2 of the back surface is

$$s_2 = r_2 - \sqrt{r_2^2 - y^2} = 240 - \sqrt{240^2 - 30^2} = 1.88 \text{ mm.}$$

Hence, the centre thickness of the lens is $t = s_1 + e - s_2 = 6.25 + 1 - 1.88 = 5.37$ mm, which should be compared with the 5.76 mm centre thickness of the spheric.

(c) We again need to calculate the sag the front surface over the $2y = 60$ mm diameter of the lens. The sag is given directly by the polynomial equation for the deformed conicoid surface; namely $x = Ay^2 + By^4 + Cy^6 + Dy^8 + Ey^{10}$, where the coefficient A is

$$A = \frac{1}{r_0 + \sqrt{r_0^2 - py^2}}$$

We evidently need the vertex radius of this front surface:

$$r_{1,0} = \frac{n_1' - n_1}{F_{1,0}} = \frac{1.6 - 1.0}{+8.30} = +0.07229 \text{ m} = +72.29 \text{ mm.}$$

Hence, the coefficient A is

$$A = \frac{1}{r_0 + \sqrt{r_0^2 - py^2}} = \frac{1}{72.29 + \sqrt{72.29^2 - 0.240 \times 30^2}}$$

$$= \frac{1}{72.29 + 70.78} = 0.0069896$$

Calculation of the front surface sag

$Ay^2 = 0.0069896 \times 30^2 = 6.2906$
$By^4 = (2.0 \times 10^{-9}) \times 30^4 = 0.00162$
$Cy^6 = (8.0 \times 10^{-11}) \times 30^6 = 0.05832$
$Dy^8 = (4.0 \times 10^{-13}) \times 30^8 = 0.26244$
$Ey^{10} = (-2.0 \times 10^{-15}) \times 30^{10} = -1.1810$

Hence, $x_1 = 6.2906 + 0.00162 + 0.05832 + 0.26244 + (-1.1810) = 5.43$ mm.
The sag of the back surface is the same as for the conicoid, since the back surface powers are identical; that is, $s_2 = 1.88$ mm. Hence, writing s_1 for x_1, the centre thickness of the lens is,

$$t = s_1 + e - s_2 = 5.43 + 1 - 1.88 = 4.55 \text{ mm.}$$

20 For the lenses in question 19, compare the sagittal heights and indicate with a diagram why this difference makes the polynomial aspheric an attractive lens for dispensing.

The sagittal height is given by $t + s_2$, see figure 4.14.

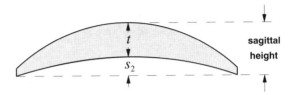

Fig. 4.14 Illustration of the sagittal height of a lens.

Evidently, the smaller the sagittal height then the less bulbous is the appearance of the lens. This is an important cosmetic requirement in spectacles since patients invariably object to lenses which appear to bulge, the implication being that the lenses are thick and their eyesight will be judged as being 'bad' by an observer.

The spheric lens   *sagittal height* $= t + s_2 = 5.76 + 3.61 = 9.37$ mm.
The conicoid lens   *sagittal height* $= t + s_2 = 5.37 + 1.88 = 7.25$ mm.
The polynomial lens   *sagittal height* $= t + s_2 = 4.55 + 1.88 = 6.43$ mm.

Note that there is an immediate reduction in sagittal due to the shallower back surface which is possible with aspheric lenses. Good oblique lens performance is maintained with this shallower form. Also, the polynomial design achieves some further saving on centre thickness due to the deformed conicoid surface, see figure 14.5.

Conicoid lens

Deformed conicoid lens (polynomial front surface)

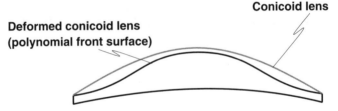

Fig. 4.15 The conicoid and deformed conicoid lenses superimposed.

Note the reduced overall thickness of the polynomial aspheric lens (deformed conicoid lens).

5   OPHTHALMIC PRISMS

Preface

In this chapter, the symbol used to indicate the base direction and magnitude of a prism is a geometric vector with a triangular arrow. Examples are shown below. Note that the length of the line indicates the power of the prism when drawn to scale, and the orientation of the line shows the base-apex line direction.

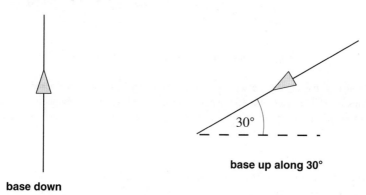

base up along 30°

base down

---

1 **A prism made in glass of refractive index 1.523 has an apical angle of 4°. What is its power in prism dioptres?**

Use the expression for deviation produced by a thin prism,

$$d = (n - 1)a.$$

Then

$$d = (n - 1)a = (1.523 - 1) \times 4° = 2.092°$$

The deviation expressed in prism dioptres is

$$100 \tan d = 100 \tan 2.092° = 3.65^\Delta.$$

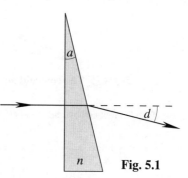

Fig. 5.1

2   A thin plano prism, made of material of refractive index 1.523, has an apical angle of
     6°. An object is apparently displaced 7.5 cm when viewed through the prism. Find the
     distance from the object to the prism.

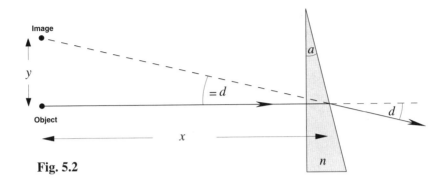

Fig. 5.2

Find the deviation produced by the prism:

$$d = (n - 1)a = (1.523 - 1) \times 6° = 3.138°$$

From the geometry of figure 5.2,

$$x = \frac{y}{\tan d} = \frac{7.5}{\tan 3.138°} = \frac{7.5}{0.0548} = 136.9 \text{ cm}.$$

---

3   A tangent scale is constructed for use at 4 metres, but is incorrectly used at 3 metres.
     When the scale is viewed through a certain prism a reading of 5^Δ is obtained. If the
     prism is made of glass of refractive index 1.523, what is its apical angle?

Since the scale is constructed for use at 4 m, its divisions are 4 cm apart. Hence, a deviation
of 5^Δ (i.e. 5 scale divisions) represents a displacement of $5 \times 4 = 20$ cm.

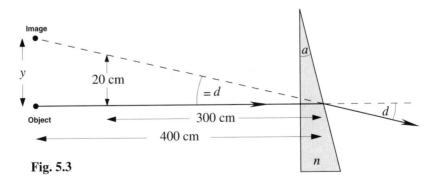

Fig. 5.3

From the definition of the prism dioptre:

$$power\,(^{\Delta}) \;=\; \frac{displacement\ of\ image\ (cm)}{distance\ from\ prism\ to\ tangent\ screen\ (m)} \;=\; \frac{20}{3} \;=\; 6.67^{\Delta}.$$

This means, of course, that the displacement at 4 m would be y, where

$$\frac{y}{4} \;=\; 6.67. \quad \text{Hence,}\ y \;=\; 4 \times 6.67 \;=\; 26.67\ \text{cm.}$$

Alternatively, the displacement at 3 m (= 300 cm) is 20 cm, from which

$$d^{\Delta} \;=\; 100 \tan d^{\circ} \;=\; 100 \times \frac{20}{300} \;=\; 6.67^{\Delta}.$$

To find the apical angle, first express d in degrees:

$$\text{Since}\ \ 100 \tan d^{\circ} = 6.67^{\Delta}, \quad d^{\circ} = \arctan \frac{6.67}{100} = 3.82^{\circ}.$$

Find the apical angle using $d = (n-1)a$. Thus,

$$a \;=\; \frac{d}{n-1} \;=\; \frac{3.82}{1.523-1} \;=\; 7.3^{\circ}.$$

---

4 An eye views an object point 30.0 cm in front of its centre of rotation. If a 6^{Δ} prism is now placed in front of the eye, 2.5 cm from its centre of rotation, find the angle through which the eye must rotate to view the object point again.

There are two stages to the solution:
(i) Find the apparent displacement of the object by the prism; this is y in figure 5.4 .
(ii) Calculate the angular subtense of this displacement at the eye's centre of rotation; θ in the figure.

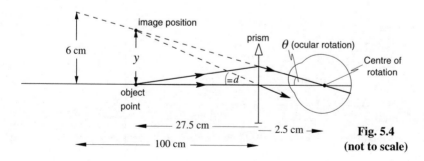

Fig. 5.4
(not to scale)

By similar triangles, $\dfrac{y}{6} = \dfrac{27.5}{100}$ from which $y = \dfrac{6 \times 27.5}{100} = 1.65$ cm.

Then $\tan \theta = \dfrac{y}{27.5 + 2.5} = \dfrac{1.65}{30} = 0.055$

from which $\theta^{\Delta} = 100 \tan \theta = 100 \times 0.055 = 5.5^{\Delta}$.

Alternatively, the expression $\theta^{\Delta} = \dfrac{P}{1 - \dfrac{s}{l}}$ may be used, where s is the distance from

the prism to the centre of rotation, and l is the distance from the prism to the object point. Note the the sign convention must be observed when using this expression: thus $l = -27.5$ cm.

Then $\theta^{\Delta} = \dfrac{P}{1 - \dfrac{s}{l}} = \dfrac{6}{1 - \dfrac{2.5}{-27.5}} = \dfrac{6}{1.09} = 5.5^{\Delta}$, as before.

---

5 An object 2 m away appears to be displaced a distance of 8 cm when viewed through a circular prism 50 mm in diameter. If the glass of which the prism is made has a refractive index of 1.62, what will be the difference in edge thickness of the prism at its base and apex?

Firstly, find the power of the prism; see figure 5.5 .

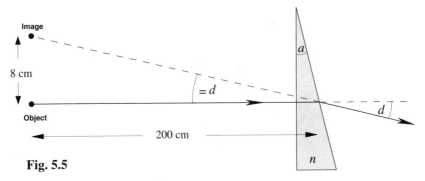

Fig. 5.5

From the figure, $d^{\Delta} = 100 \tan d^{\circ} = 100 \times \dfrac{8}{200} = 4^{\Delta}$.

We can also arrive at the power of the prism by using the definition $P^{\Delta} = \dfrac{y}{x} \dfrac{\text{cm}}{\text{m}}$

where y is the displacement and x is the distance from the object to the prism.

Thus, $P = \dfrac{y}{x} = \dfrac{8}{2} \left(\dfrac{\text{cm}}{\text{m}}\right) = 4^{\Delta}$.

We now use the prism edge thickness difference formula. The diameter d of the round shaped prism is shown in the section illustrated in figure 5.6 . g is the difference between the apex and base edge thicknesses, the apex being knife-edge here. Then,

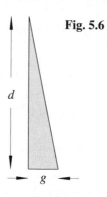

Fig. 5.6

$$g = \frac{Pd}{100\,(n-1)}$$

$$= \frac{4 \times 50}{100 \times (1.62 - 1)}$$

$$= 3.23 \text{ mm.}$$

Note: In the prism thickness difference formula, P is the prism power and d is the diameter of the prism. Do not confuse the use of d for deviation and diameter.

---

6   **A circular prism of 45 mm diameter has a difference in edge thickness between its base and apex of 4 mm. It is made of glass of refractive index 1.523 . What will be the apparent displacement of an object 2 m away when viewed through this prism?**

Find the power of the prism from the expression for prism thickness difference (see above).

Thus, $P = \dfrac{100\,g\,(n-1)}{d} = \dfrac{100 \times 4 \times (1.523 - 1)}{45} = 4.65^{\wedge}.$

Find the displacement from figure 5.7 :

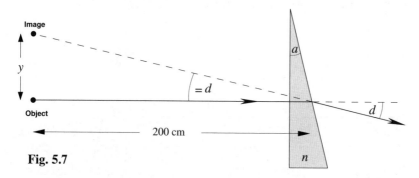

Fig. 5.7

The displacement (y) of the image is

$$y = 200 \tan d = 200 \times \frac{4.65}{100} = 9.30 \text{ cm (having used } 100 \tan d = 4.65^{\triangle}).$$

Or, using the definition of prism power:

$$P = \frac{y}{x}, \quad \text{so} \quad y = Px = 4.65 \times 200 = 9.30 \text{ cm.}$$

7   A tangent scale is 150 cm from a thin prism. It appears to be displaced 6 cm when viewed through the prism. The prism is circular with a diameter of 40 mm and the difference in edge thickness at its base and apex is 3 mm. What is the the refractive index of the glass from which the prism is made?

Find the power of the prism.

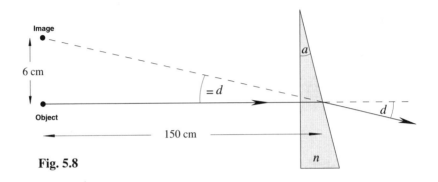

Fig. 5.8

$$\tan d° = \frac{6}{150} = 0.04, \text{ from which, } d^\Delta = 100 \tan d° = 100 \times 0.04 = 4^\Delta.$$

(Alternatively, $P = \frac{y}{x} = \frac{6}{1.5} = 4^\Delta$.)

Find the refractive index from the prism thickness difference formula, $g = \dfrac{Pd}{100\,(n-1)}$.

That is, $n = \dfrac{Pd}{100g} + 1 = \dfrac{4 \times 40}{100 \times 3} + 1 = 1.53$.

---

8   **What single prism is equivalent to 5^Δ base down and 2^Δ base out for a left eye?**

The steps for a graphical method of compounding prisms are as follows:
1. Choose a suitable scale, say 1 cm $\equiv 1^\Delta$.
2. From a common origin, O, construct the prism vectors to scale along their stated directions.
3. Complete the rectangle and construct the diagonal from the origin.
4. Measure the diagonal for length and orientation.
   N.B. The base direction must be stated in standard notation.

In figure 5.9, by measurement, the resultant (OR) is 5.4^Δ base down along $112°$.

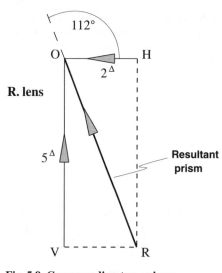

Alternatively, the resultant may be found by calculation:

$$OR = \sqrt{OV^2 + OH^2} = \sqrt{5^2 + 2^2} = 5.4$$

and $\tan VOR = \dfrac{VR}{OV} = \dfrac{2}{5} = 0.4$

so, $\angle VOR = \arctan 0.4 = 21.8°$

which gives a standard notation angle of

$$21.8° + 90° = 111.8°.$$

By calculation, the resultant is therefore

5.4^Δ base down $111.8°$.

Fig. 5.9 Compounding two prisms.
5^Δ base down and 2^Δ base out.

An alternative to the 'parallelogram of prisms' (in this case a rectangle, figure 5.9) is the triangle of prisms; that is, a vector triangle. This is exactly the same as the construction of a triangle of forces in mechanics. Forces and thin prisms have both magnitude and direction, and they can therefore be modelled by geometric vectors (or simply vectors, for short). The triangle of prisms is shown in figure 5.10, drawn on the same scale as figure 5.9 . Either figure 5.10(a) or (b) will do. The resultant is AC in figure 5.10(a) and DE in figure 5.10(b). The calculation is left to the student.

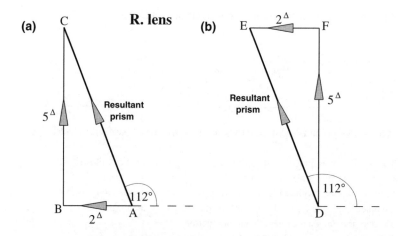

Fig. 5.10 Compounding two prisms, 5^Δ base down and 2^Δ base out,
using a vector triangle.

42

9   **Find the horizontal and vertical components of the plano prism R. 5^Δ base down $30°$.**

For resolving prisms with oblique base directions into their horizontal and vertical components, the graphical method is as follows:
1. Choose a suitable scale, say 1 cm ≡ 1^Δ.
2. From the origin, construct the given prism vector OR to scale along its stated base direction.
3. Drop perpendiculars RV and RH onto the vertical and horizontal meridians, respectively.
4. Measure the distances OV and OH which represent the component prisms required.

In figure 5.11(a), by measurement, OH is 4.35^Δ base out and OV is 2.5^Δ base down.

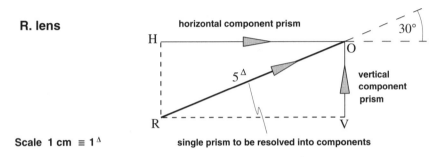

R. lens

Scale 1 cm ≡ 1^Δ

Fig. 5.11(a) Resolving a prism, 5^Δ base down $30°$, to find its horizontal and vertical components. Note that by the 'parallelogram of prisms' method, the prism vector arrows end up either pointing towards the origin or away from it.

Alternatively, the components can be found by calculation:

OH = OR cos 30° = 5 × 0.8660 = 4.33^Δ and OV = OR sin 30° = 5 × 0.5 = 2.5^Δ.

That is, 4.33^Δ base out and 2.5^Δ base down, the base directions being obtained from the vectors in figure 5.11 .

Again, a vector triangle model, rather than a rectangular one, may be used.

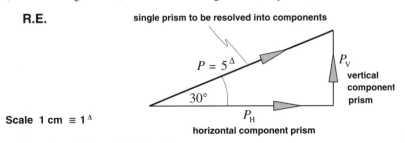

R.E.

Scale 1 cm ≡ 1^Δ

Fig. 5.11(b) Vector triangle alternative for problem 9.

10 **Find the resultant of placing the following prisms one in front of the other in a trial frame before a left eye.** 4^Δ **base up 40° and** 5^Δ **base up 110°.**

The graphical method for compounding prisms of any angle is very similar to that given in question 5.8 for compounding two prisms at right angles. However, the third step should read: *Complete the parallelogram and construct the diagonal from the origin.*

In figure 5.12, the prisms to be compounded are drawn to the origin O. That is, 4^Δ is modelled by a vector 4 cm long at 40° to the horizontal, with its vector arrow indicating the prism base direction is UP 40°. Similarly, the 5^Δ base UP 110° is shown as a 5 cm line with the vector arrow upwards along the 110° direction. The resultant is found by constructing the parallelogram, as stated in the paragraph above, whence the diagonal OR represents the resultant prism.

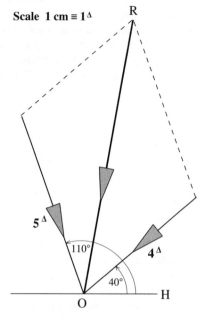

Scale 1 cm ≡ 1^Δ

Fig. 5.12

Hence, by measurement in figure 5.12, the resultant is OR = 7.4 cm, which means that the resultant is 7.4^Δ. Since all the vector arrows point towards the origin O, the resultant prism has its base direction UP at the angle HOR. By measurement, $\angle$HOR = 79.5°.

Alternative method 1
We can resolve each oblique prism into its horizontal and vertical components as shown in question 5.9 . The horizontal components are then added to obtain the horizontal component of the resultant, and a similar process will find the vertical component of the resultant. The method is shown in figure 5.13 .

Right Eye

Fig. 5.13

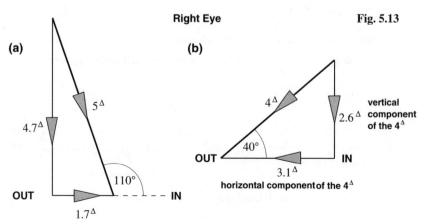

44

By measurements in figure 5.13, the components of the two prisms are:

Vertical components 4.7^Δ base up and 2.6^Δ base up
Horizontal components 3.1^Δ base out and 1.7^Δ base in.

These add together to give the horizontal and vertical components of the resultant:

$$4.7^\Delta \text{ base up} + 2.6^\Delta \text{ base up} = 7.3^\Delta \text{ base up}$$

and 3.1^Δ base out + 1.7^Δ base in = 1.4^Δ base out.

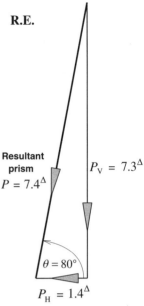

**Resultant
prism**
$P = 7.4^\Delta$

$P_V = 7.3^\Delta$

$\theta = 80°$

$P_H = 1.4^\Delta$

Fig. 5.14 Scale 1 cm $\equiv 1^\Delta$

The resultant is found by compounding the 7.3^Δ base up and the 1.4^Δ base out; see figure 5.14 . Either a scale diagram or trigonometry may be used to determine the resultant prism value and the 80° angle. Figure 5.14 is a vector addition, drawn to scale, so the values shown therein may be verified by measurement. For the calculation of the resultant, calling the vertical component P_V, the horizontal component P_H, the resultant P, and the angle (θ) the resultant makes with the horizontal, then

$$P = \sqrt{P_H^2 + P_V^2} = \sqrt{1.4^2 + 7.3^2} = 7.4^\Delta$$

and $\tan \theta = \dfrac{P_V}{P_H} = \dfrac{7.3}{1.4} = 5.2$, so $\theta = \arctan 5.2 = 79°$.

Alternative method 2

We can solve the triangle of prisms trigonometrically; see figure 5.15 .
AC is the resultant prism (note that both the resultant, and the components CB and BA combined, 'lead' from the point C to the point A).

Now, $\angle ABE = 180° - \angle BAD = 180° - 40° = 140°$,

and $\angle ABC = 360° - (\angle ABE + \angle CBE)$
$= 360° - (140° + 110°)$
$= 110°$.

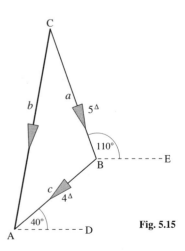

C

b

a

5^Δ

$110°$

B ----- E

c

4^Δ

$40°$

A ----- D

Fig. 5.15

We can now use the cosine rule to find AC, designated b in figure 5.15 .
So, $b^2 = a^2 + c^2 - 2ac \cos \angle ABC$
$= 5^2 + 4^2 - 2 \times 5 \times 4 \times \cos 110°$
$= 54.68$
whence $b = \sqrt{(54.68)} = 7.39$. This is the magnitude

of the resultant prism. We need to find the angle CAD where
$$\angle CAD = \angle CAB + \angle BAD = \angle CAB + 40°$$
Clearly, we must find $\angle CAB$. Using the sine rule on triangle ABC,

$$\frac{\sin A}{a} = \frac{\sin B}{b} \quad \text{or} \quad \sin A = \frac{a}{b}\sin B = \frac{5}{7.39}\sin 110° = \frac{5}{7.39} \times 0.9397 = 0.6358$$

giving $A = \angle CAB = \arcsin 0.6458 = 39.48°$.

So, $\angle CAD = \angle CAB + \angle BAD = 39.48° + 40° = 79.48°$. This is the angle the resultant prism makes with the horizontal. By measurement from figure 5.12, we found this to be 79.5°.

Yet a third variant is to draw figure 5.15 to scale and measure AC and $\angle CAD$. This would be a relatively simple method in an examination question.

---

11 **The following prisms are to be included in a prescription for a pair of spectacle lenses:**
   R. 2.5^Δ base up 150° and L. 3.5^Δ base down 120°.
These prisms are to be equally divided between the two eyes. What will be the single resultant effect in each eye?

Resolve each prism into its horizontal and vertical components; see figure 5.16 .

Fig. 5.16

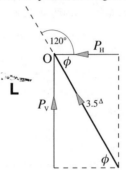

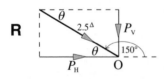

By calculation:

   Right $P_V = 2.5 \sin \theta = 2.5 \sin 30° = 2.5 \times 0.5 = 1.25^\Delta$ base up.
            $P_H = 2.5 \cos \theta = 2.5 \cos 30° = 2.5 \times 0.866 = 2.17^\Delta$ base out.

   Left $P_V = 3.5 \sin \phi = 3.5 \sin 60° = 3.5 \times 0.866 = 3.03^\Delta$ base down.
            $P_H = 3.5 \cos \phi = 3.5 \cos 60° = 3.5 \times 0.5 = 1.75^\Delta$ base out.

Therefore, the differential prismatic effect is:

   Vertically, $1.25 + 3.03 = 4.28^\Delta$ base down left (or base up right)
   Horizontally, $2.17 + 1.75 = 3.92^\Delta$ base out right or left.

Split equally between the two eyes, these prisms are:
   R. 2.14^Δ base up / 1.96^Δ base out   and   L. 2.14^Δ base down / 1.96^Δ base out.

Compound these horizontal and vertical prisms in each eye to obtain the resultant: see figure 5.17 .

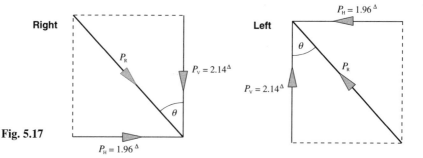

Fig. 5.17

In each case, the magnitude of the resultant prism (P_R) is the same, but the base directions are opposed.

$$P_R = \sqrt{P_H^2 + P_V^2} = \sqrt{2.14^2 + 1.96^2} = 2.9^\Delta.$$

The base direction can be found from figure 5.17,

$$\tan \theta = \frac{1.96}{2.14} = 0.9159, \quad \text{so} \quad \theta = \arctan 0.9159 = 42.5°.$$

In standard notation, the base direction is $42.5° + 90° = 132.5°$.

An alternative method

The single relative prism before the right eye, say, can be found directly by using the vector method. Students familiar with relative velocities will recognise the procedure.

Relative to the left eye, the prismatic effect in the right eye can be found by adding 3.5^Δ base up along 120° to each eye. This negates the prism in the left eye. The prism can now be regarded as being entirely before the right eye, and this is shown in figure 5.18 as the resultant AC.

AC represents 5.8^Δ base up 132.5° and this can be split as:

    R. 2.9^Δ base up 132.5°

and L. 2.9^Δ base down 132.5°.

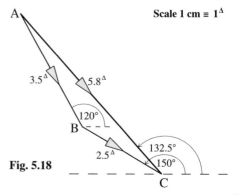

Fig. 5.18

12 A rotary prism device is placed in the cell of a trial frame with its zero setting at 150°. Each prism is $6^\triangle$. The prisms are then rotated 25° from the zero position. What is the power and base setting of the resultant?

In figure 5.19, the prisms in their zero setting (that is, with their bases opposed) are shown as dashed lines. Each prism is then rotated towards the other through 25°. The resultant OR can be found either by measurement or by calculation.

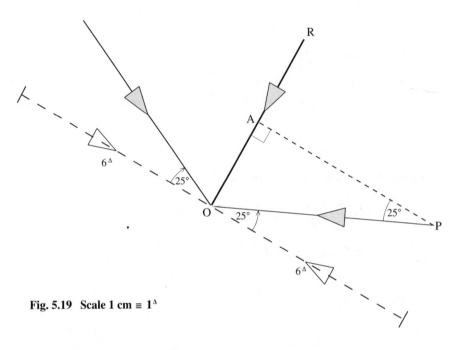

Fig. 5.19 Scale 1 cm ≡ $1^\triangle$

By measurement,   OR = $5^\triangle$ base up 60°.

By calculation,   OA = AR = OP sin 25° = 6 × 0.4226 = $2.536^\triangle$.

Therefore   OR = 2 AR = 2 × 2.536 = $5.072^\triangle$.

From the figure, it should be apparent that ∠ROP = 65°, which places OR at right-angles to the 150° meridian. Hence, OR lies along the 60° meridian.

13 **A 4^Δ plano-prism is placed base up 30°. What are its components along the 60° and 150° meridians?**

In figure 5.20, BA represents 4^Δ base up along 30°. BC is its component along 150°, and CA is its component along 60°. Measurement gives: 2^Δ base down 150° and 3.5^Δ base up 60°.

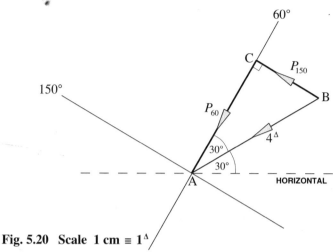

Fig. 5.20 Scale 1 cm $\equiv$ 1$^\Delta$

By calculation: $\angle CAB = 60° - 30° = 30°$ and $\angle CBA = 60°$.

$\angle ACB = 90°$, by construction.

From triangle ABC, the prism component along 150°, P_{150}, is

$$P_{150} = BC = AB \sin \angle CAB = 4 \sin 30° = 2^\Delta \text{ base down } 150°.$$

The base direction was obtained, as usual by inspection of the vector triangle ABC.

The prism component along 60° is:

$$P_{60} = CA = AB \cos \angle CAB = 4 \cos 30° = 3.5^\Delta \text{ base up } 60°.$$

49

14 **Three thin prisms are placed in contact before a right eye. The prisms are:**
   (a) 2^Δ base out,   (b) 1^Δ base down,   and (c) 2^Δ base down 120°.
Find the resultant prism.

First method

We resolve each prism into horizontal and vertical components:
(a) 2^Δ base out (no vertical component),
(b) 1^Δ base down (no horizontal component),
(c)   Figure 5.21 shows the 2^Δ base down 120°. CA represents this prism, and CB and BA are its horizontal and vertical components, respectively.

Now, BA $= $ CA $\sin 60° = 2 \times 0.866$
          $= 1.732^\Delta$ base down.

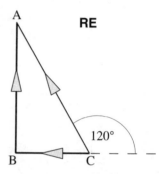

RE

and   CB $= $ CA $\cos 60° = 2 \times 0.500$
          $= 1^\Delta$ base in.

(Base directions from the construction of the vector triangle.)

<u>Add together all horizontal components</u>

   2^Δ base out $+ 1^\Delta$ base in $= 1^\Delta$ base out.

Fig. 5.21

This is the horizontal component of the resultant. Now add together the vertical components:

1^Δ base down $+ 1.732^\Delta$ base down $= 2.732^\Delta$ base down.

We find the resultant by compounding its horizontal component, 1^Δ base out, with its vertical component, 2.732^Δ base down.   Figure 5.22 shows the vector triangle.

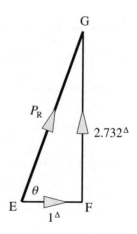

The resultant is

$$P_R = \sqrt{EF^2 + FG^2} = \sqrt{1^2 + 2.732^2} = 2.91^\Delta.$$

Its base-apex setting is

$$\theta = \arctan \frac{2.732}{1} = 69.9°.$$

So, the resultant prism is $P_R = 2.91^\Delta$ base down 69.9°, the base direction being obtained from the rules of vector addition in figure 5.22.

Fig. 5.22

Second method

Join all three prisms 'head-to-tail' as in figure 5.23, drawn to the scale 1 cm $\equiv 1^\Delta$.

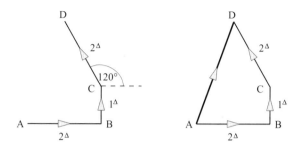

Fig. 5.23   Scale: 1 cm$\equiv 1^\Delta$

The resultant is found by joining AD. By measurement, the resultant is

$$P_R \;=\; AD \;=\; 2.9^\Delta \qquad \text{and} \qquad \angle DAB \;=\; 70°.$$

6   PRISMATIC EFFECTS

Preface: As in the previous chapter, the same symbol, a triangle, is used to indicate the base direction of any prismatic effect.

For example:

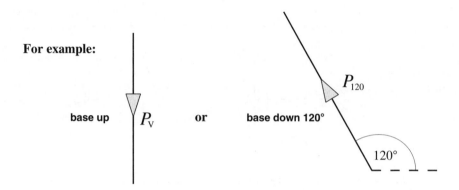

base up P_V **or**   base down 120° P_{120}

120°

The symbol used for decentration is an arrow indicating the direction of movement of the optical centre during the process of decentration.

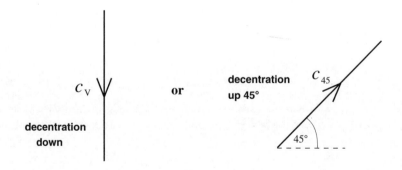

c_V **or**   decentration up 45° c_{45}

decentration down   45°

Note the use of P for prismatic effect and c for decentration, with subscripts indicating the direction. For example, the subscript v for vertical and 45 for 45°, and so on.

1   Calculate the vertical and horizontal prismatic effects encountered by a subject when viewing through a point 8 mm below and 3 mm in from the optical centre of a +6.00 DS lens before his right eye.

Use Prentice's Rule $(P = cF$ or $P = c\,|F\,|)$ to find the magnitude of the prismatic effects.

The base directions of the prismatic effect induced by a lens can be obtained with the help of various versions of a diagrammatic representation of the lens. An attempt should be made to visualise the lens, and figure 6.1 is an example of the kind of diagram which may be found useful initially.

To obtain the base direction of a prismatic effect it is a simple matter of observing where the optical centre of the lens lies in relation to the visual point.

Note: (i)   With a *positive* lens, the base of the prism is always *towards* the optical centre; see figure 6.1 .

      (ii)   With a *negative lens* it is always *away* from the optical centre; see figure 6.2 .

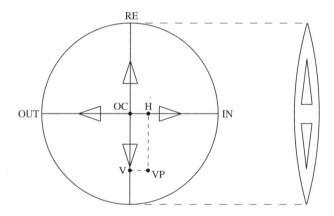

Fig. 6.1   Illustration of the prismatic effect at a point on a positive lens.

The visual point (VP) is projected onto the vertical and horizontal meridians at the points V and H, respectively. It can be seen that since the optical centre (OC) is directly above V, the base direction of the induced vertical prismatic effect is UP. Similarly, the optical centre is out in relation to H, therefore the base direction of the induced horizontal prismatic effect is OUT.

Hence, the vertical prismatic effect (P_V) is given by

$$P_V \;=\; c_V\,|F_V| \;=\; 0.8 \times 6 \;=\; 4.8^\Delta \text{ base up,}$$

and the horizontal prismatic effect (P_H) is given by

$$P_H \;=\; c_H\,|F_H| \;=\; 0.3 \times 6 \;=\; 1.8^\Delta \text{ base out.}$$

2 At what point on a –3.25 DS lens will a subject's left eye encounter the prismatic effects 2.75$^\Delta$ base down and 0.75$^\Delta$ base in?

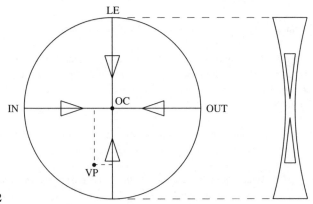

Fig. 6.2

The distance from the optical centre (OC) to the the visual point (VP) is calculated using Prentice's Rule which transposes into $c = P/|F|$. The position of the visual point is stated in relation to the optical centre, and is perhaps best obtained by visualising the lens as in figure 6.2 .

By drawing in the symbols representing the base directions on the vertical and horizontal meridians (this is a minus lens and the prism bases are *away* from the optical centre) it is clear that in order to obtain prism base directions DOWN and IN, the visual point must be BELOW and IN from the optical centre.

(Note: the decentration c in Prentice's Rule must be in centimetres.)

Then, $c_V = \dfrac{P_V}{|F_V|} = \dfrac{2.75}{3.25} = 0.85$ cm = 8.5 mm below the optical centre

and $c_H = \dfrac{P_H}{|F_H|} = \dfrac{0.75}{3.25} = 0.23$ cm = 2.3 mm in from the optical centre.

---

3 Find the decentration required to produce 2$^\Delta$ base down and 3$^\Delta$ base in on the lens L. +8.00 DS.

The amount of decentration is obtained using Prentice's Rule, $P = c|F|$, rearranged to give $c = P/|F|$.

The direction of decentration can be found in a number of ways. Again, a diagram of the lens can be useful to see where the visual point must lie in relation to the optical centre. In this question, base down and base in effects are required, and it can be seen from figure 6.3 that, for these prismatic effects, the visual point must lie somewhere in the upper right quadrant.

It is necessary to determine what movement of the optical centre will result in the visual point being placed in this position. (It is assumed that initially the visual point and the optical centre coincide.) From figure 6.3, it is evident that the optical centre has been moved downwards and inwards from VP.

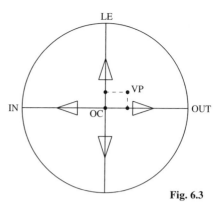

Fig. 6.3

Alternatively, the rule which gives the direction of the decentration is as follows:

*If the lens (or meridian) is **positive**, decentre in the **same** direction as the prism base.*
*If the lens (or meridian) is **negative**, decentre in the **opposite** direction to the prism base.*

$$\text{Thus,} \quad c_V = \frac{P_V}{|F_V|} = \frac{2}{8} = 0.25 \text{ cm} = 2.5 \text{ mm downwards}$$

$$\text{and} \quad c_H = \frac{P_H}{|F_H|} = \frac{3}{8} = 0.375 \text{ cm} = 3.75 \text{ mm inwards.}$$

---

4 Find the vertical and horizontal prismatic effects produced when the lens R. +2.00 / −5.00 x 180   is decentred 4 mm upwards and 5 mm inwards.

A sph/cyl prescription is best dealt with by determining its principal powers and applying Prentice's Rule to each meridian separately. The base directions of the prismatic effects can be obtained by combining the power diagram with the base direction diagram as in figure 6.4.

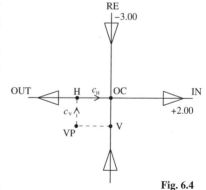

Fig. 6.4

Since in this question the lens has been decentred *upwards* and *inwards*, the point (VP) at which the prismatic effect is to be found is *down* and *out* from the optical centre (OC). The visual point VP projects onto the horizontal meridian at the point H. At this point the prism base direction is IN. At the point V, where the visual point VP projects onto the vertical meridian, the base direction is DOWN.

$$\text{Thus} \quad P_V = c_V |F_V| = 0.4 \times 3 = 1.2^\Delta \text{ base down,}$$

$$\text{and} \quad P_H = c_H |F_H| = 0.5 \times 2 = 1.0^\Delta \text{ base in.}$$

5 Calculate the horizontal and vertical decentration required to produce the following prescription: **L. −2.50 / +5.50 x 180 / 2△ base in / 1.5△ base up.**

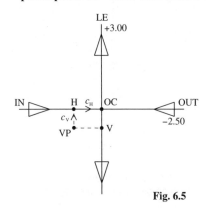

LE
+3.00

IN — H c_H OC — OUT
c_V
VP – – – V
−2.50

Fig. 6.5

Determine the principal powers and apply Prentice's Rule to each meridian in turn.

The direction of decentration can be determined by inspection of a base direction diagram such as figure 6.5. Alternatively, the rules of decentration can be applied (see question 6.3).

From the figure, in order that there should be base IN and base UP effect at the visual point (VP), the optical centre must be moved upwards and outwards.

Hence, $\quad c_V \;=\; \dfrac{P_V}{|F_V|} \;=\; \dfrac{1.5}{3} \;=\; 0.5\text{ cm} \;=\; 5\text{ mm upwards}$

and $\quad c_H \;=\; \dfrac{P_H}{|F_H|} \;=\; \dfrac{2}{2.5} \;=\; 0.8\text{ cm} \;=\; 8\text{ mm outwards.}$

---

6 Find the minimum diameter of the circular uncut from which the following prescription can be obtained by decentration. The finished lens size is to be 48 mm round.
R. +5.75 / +1.00 x 90 / 2△ base in / 1.5△ base up.

Calculate the amount and direction of decentration required using the method shown in questions 6.3 and 6.5. In this case, however, a single resultant decentration will be needed; see figure 6.7. Figure 6.6 indicates that the visual point (VP) will be down and out from the optical centre in order to produce base in and base up prismatic effects. Using Prentice's Rule, to find the decentration relative to VP, the necessary decentration components are:

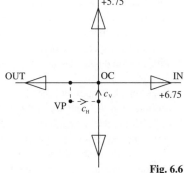

+5.75

OUT — OC — IN
c_V
VP $\rightarrow$ –
c_H
+6.75

Fig. 6.6

$$c_V \;=\; \frac{P_V}{|F_V|} \;=\; \frac{1.5}{5.75} \;=\; 0.26\text{ cm} \;=\; 2.6\text{ mm upwards}$$

and $\quad c_H \;=\; \dfrac{P_H}{|F_H|} \;=\; \dfrac{2}{6.75} \;=\; 0.30\text{ cm} \;=\; 3.0\text{ mm inwards.}$

The single resultant decentration, c, and its direction can be found from figure 6.7:

$$c = \sqrt{c_H^2 + c_V^2} = \sqrt{3^2 + 2.6^2} = 4.0 \text{ mm.}$$

and $\quad \tan \theta = \dfrac{2.6}{3} = 0.867$

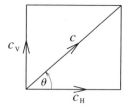

so $\theta = 40.9°$.

Fig. 6.7

That is, the single resultant decentration is 4.0 mm up 40.9°.

The minimum size uncut (*MSU*) is obtained from

$$MSU = lens \ size + (2 \times decentration)$$

$$= 48 + (2 \times 4.0)$$

$$= 56 \text{ mm.}$$

---

7   **The lens +2.50 / –5.50 x 180 is decentred 8 mm up 60° before a right eye. Calculate the single resultant prismatic effect which will be produced.**

Before the calculation of prismatic effects can begin, the oblique decentration must be resolved into its vertical and horizontal components; that is, along the principal meridians as shown in figure 6.8 .

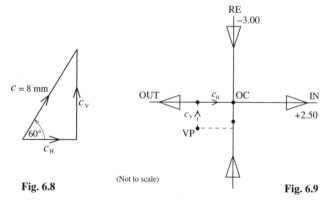

Fig. 6.8   (Not to scale)   **Fig. 6.9**

From figure 6.8,   the vertical decentration is $c_V = 8 \sin 60° = 6.9$ mm upwards
and the horizontal decentration is $c_H = 8 \cos 60° = 4.0$ mm inwards.

Since the lens has been decentred upwards and inwards, relative to the visual point (VP), the point at which the prismatic effect is to be found is down and out from the optical centre; see figure 6.9 . Using Prentice's Rule, we have

$$P_V = c_V |F_V| = 0.69 \times 3 = 2.1^\triangle \text{ base down,}$$

$$\text{and} \quad P_H = c_H |F_H| = 0.4 \times 2.5 = 1.0^\triangle \text{ base in.}$$

To obtain the single resultant prismatic effect, these prisms must now be compounded. Using figure 6.10,

$$P = \sqrt{P_H{}^2 + P_V{}^2} = \sqrt{1^2 + 2.1^2} = 2.3^\triangle$$

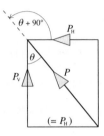

$$\text{and} \quad \tan \theta = \frac{P_H}{P_V} = \frac{1.0}{2.1} = 0.4762$$

so that $\theta = 25.5°$.

In standard notation, the base direction of the resultant prism (P) is $25.5° + 90° = 115.5°$.

Fig. 6.10

Hence, the single resultant is $2.3^\triangle$ base down 115.5°.

---

8 **Find the vertical and horizontal prismatic effects at a point 7 mm below and 3 mm in from the optical centre of the lens: R. −2.50 / −3.25 x 70.**

When determining the prismatic effect produced by a lens in which the principal meridians are oblique, there are at least two graphical methods which may be used, and it is possible also to obtain the result by calculation. This question will be worked using two of the most common graphical solutions. The first construction uses the method in which the prismatic effect due to the sphere and cylinder are considered separately. It is followed by the construction in which the lens is considered as a crossed cylinder.

First method *Prismatic effect due to sphere and cylinder considered separately.*

(i) Prismatic effect due to *sphere*

The sphere power is −2.50 D and the point on the lens is 7 mm below and 3 mm in from the optical centre; see figure 6.11(a). For the purpose of using Prentice's Rule, we can consider the optical centre OC has been decentred 3 mm out and 7 mm up from the visual point (VP) at which the prismatic effect is to be determined. Note that at VP the diagram indicates that there will be base in and base down component prisms.

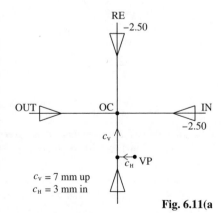

Fig. 6.11(a

58

Hence, using Prentice's Rule,

$$P_V = c_V |F_V| = 0.7 \times 2.50 = 1.75^\Delta \text{ base down,}$$

and $\quad P_H = c_H |F_H| = 0.3 \times 2.50 = 0.75^\Delta \text{ base in.}$

(ii) Prismatic effect due to *cylinder*

Refer to figure 6.11(b)

Construct the vertical and horizontal meridians and the cylinder axis (70°).

With a convenient scale, say 1 cm ≡ 1 mm, locate the point Q at which the prismatic effect is to be found. In this particular case, 7 mm down and 3 mm in from the optical centre O.

Drop a perpendicular from this point Q onto the axis. This gives *c*, the resultant decentration.

Resolve *c* into its vertical and horizontal components, c_V and c_H. By measurement, and referring to the scale, $c_V = 1.8$ mm and $c_H = 4.9$ mm.

Using the values of c_V and c_H found above, calculate the vertical and horizontal prismatic effects due to the cylinder.

Since this is a minus cylinder, the base direction of the induced prismatic effect is perpendicularly *away* from the axis; that is, in this case the base direction is *down* (and *in*) along 160°. This gives vertical and horizontal prismatic effects of:

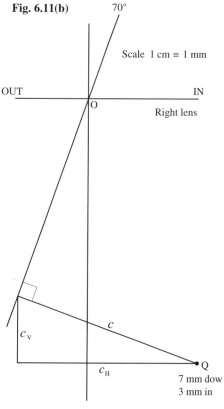

Fig. 6.11(b)   70°

Scale 1 cm ≡ 1 mm

OUT   IN

Right lens

7 mm dow
3 mm in

$$P_V = c_V |F_V| = 0.18 \times 3.25 = 0.59^\Delta \text{ base down,}$$

and $\quad P_H = c_H |F_H| = 0.49 \times 3.25 = 1.59^\Delta \text{ base in.}$

Now add together the vertical and horizontal prismatic effects due to the sphere and cylinder:

P_V due to the sphere	1.75^Δ base down	P_H due to the sphere	0.75^Δ base in
P_V due to the cylinder	0.59^Δ base down	P_H due to the cylinder	1.59^Δ base in
	2.34^Δ base down		2.34^Δ base in

59

Alternative method of determining the prismatic effect due to the cylinder

This is a slight variation on the previous method; here the single prismatic effect is found and then the horizontal and vertical components are determined.

Construct the vertical and horizontal meridians and the cylinder axis; see figure 6.12. Using a 1 cm ≡ 1 mm scale, locate the point at which the prismatic effect is to be found (7 mm below and 3 mm in from the optical centre). Drop a perpendicular from this point onto the axis and measure its length: $c = 5.2$ mm.

Applying Prentice's Rule to the cylinder, whose power is perpendicular to the axis,

$$P = c\,|F_{\text{cyl}}| = 0.52 \times 3.25 = 1.7^{\Delta}.$$

This is a minus cylinder and the prism base is *away* from the axis. That is, the resultant is 1.7^{Δ} base down 160°. This can be seen in the schematic bottom part of the diagram.

Resolve this oblique prism into its vertical and horizontal components; see figure 6.13. This can be done either by scale diagram or by trigonometry; we shall choose the latter. There is no need to draw figure 6.13 to scale.

Thus $P_V = P \sin 20° = 1.7 \times 0.342$
$\qquad\qquad = 0.58^{\Delta}$

and $P_H = P \cos 20° = 1.7 \times 0.937$
$\qquad\qquad = 1.59^{\Delta}.$

The slight difference in the value of P_V is due to the negligible inaccuracy of the scale drawing method. The rest of the solution follows the same method as before.

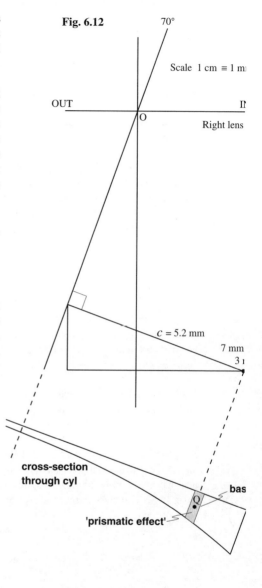

Fig. 6.12   70°

Scale 1 cm ≡ 1 mm

OUT   IN

O   Right lens

$c = 5.2$ mm

7 mm
3 mm

cross-section through cyl

base

'prismatic effect'

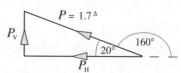

$P = 1.7^{\Delta}$

P_V

P_H

20°   160°

Fig. 6.13 P is the prismatic effect due to the cylinder.

Second method   *Prismatic effect due to the lens being considered as crossed cylinders*

Construct the vertical and horizontal meridians and the principal meridians of the lens; see figure 6.14(a).

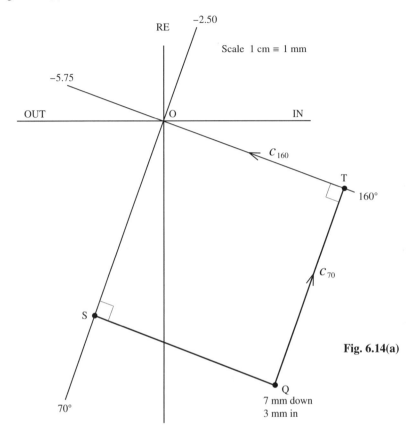

Fig. 6.14(a)

Using a convenient scale, here 1 cm ≡ 1 mm, locate the point Q at which the prismatic effect is to be found.   Q is 7 mm below and 3 mm in from the optical centre O.   Drop perpendiculars from Q onto each principal meridian, meeting them at S and T. Measure OS and OT.   From the construction, OS = 5.5 mm and OT = 5.2 mm.

Calculate the prismatic effects which will be produced along each principal meridian by the distances OS (or TQ) and OT. Note that these can be regarded as decentration components, c_{70} and c_{160}, as though the optical centre was initially at the fixed point Q in space, but has been decentred to the position shown at O.

Thus, $P_{70} = c_{70} \, |F_{70}| = 0.55 \times 2.5 = 1.375^\triangle$ base down 70°.

(The base direction is down the 70° meridian because this is a minus meridian and the point Q is below the optical centre, as measured along this meridian.   A sketch of the shape of lens section along 70° will show this.)

61

Next, $P_{160} = c_{160} |F_{160}| = 0.52 \times 5.75 = 2.99^\triangle$ base down 160°.

The determination of the base direction is similar to that for the 70° meridian. These prismatic effects are shown schematically in figure 6.14(b) below.

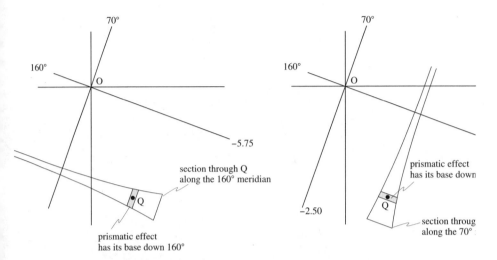

Fig. 6.14(b) **Sections through the point Q parallel to the principal meridians 160° and 70°. This sort of schematic diagram allows one to observe the base directions of the prismatic effects, from which one can deduce some rule for their determination. For example, if the optical centre can be considered decentred up on a minus me (say c_{70} in figure 6.14(a)), then the prismatic effect will be base down that meric as shown on the right above.**

Having obtained the prismatic effects P_{70} and P_{160}, now resolve these prisms into their vertical and horizontal components; see figure 6.15.

Construct the vertical and horizontal meridians and the principal meridians. Using a convenient scale, here $1'' \equiv 1^\triangle$, mark off the prism components $P_{70} = 1.375^\triangle$ base down 70° and $P_{160} = 2.99^\triangle$ base down 160° along the principal meridians in their stated directions, and complete the rectangle OPRQ. (Note: OR is the single resultant prismatic effect P_R, although it is not required here.) Drop perpendiculars from R onto the vertical and horizontal meridians, meeting them at V and H, respectively. OV is the vertical prismatic effect and OH the horizontal prismatic effect.

By measurement, using the scale,

$OV = 2.33^\triangle$ base down   and $OH = 2.35^\triangle$ base in.

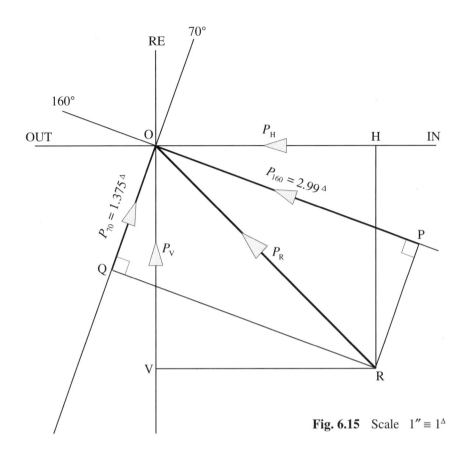

Fig. 6.15   Scale $1'' \equiv 1^\triangle$

---

9   **What prismatic effect, expressed vertically and horizontally, is produced when the lens +3.00 / +4.00 x 120 is decentred 3 mm in and 4 mm down in front of a left eye?**

This question will be answered graphically using methods set out in question 6.8 .

NB   The lens in this question has been decentred; that is, the optical centre has been moved, in this case, downwards and inwards. The point at which the prismatic effect is to be found is therefore upwards and outwards from the optical centre.

First method   *Prismatic effect due to sphere and cylinder considered separately.*

AD is the vertical decentration and DO the horizontal decentration as far as the sphere is concerned, so the horizontal and vertical prismatic effects due to the sphere are

$$P_V = c_V |F_{sph}| = 0.4 \times 3 = 1.2^\triangle \text{ base down}$$

and

$$P_H = c_H |F_{sph}| = 0.3 \times 3 = 0.9^\triangle \text{ base in.}$$

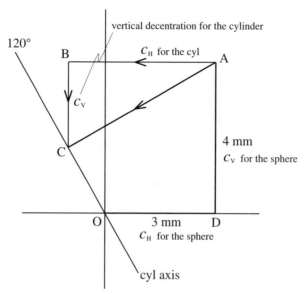

Fig. 6.16   Scale 1 cm ≡ 1 mm

Prismatic effect due to the cylinder:

Note that CA can be considered as the decentration as far as the cylindrical power is concerned. This distance has components AB and BC which are shown as c_H and c_V in figure 6.16. (For the step-by step method, see question 8.)

By measurement, $c_V = 2.3$ mm and $c_H = 4$ mm. Hence,

$$P_V = c_V \, |F_{cyl}| = 0.23 \times 4 = 0.92^\Delta \text{ base down}$$

and

$$P_H = c_H \, |F_{cyl}| = 0.4 \times 4 = 1.6^\Delta \text{ base in.}$$

Adding the prismatic effects due to the sphere and those due to the cylinder, we have:

$P_{V, \, sph} = 1.20^\Delta$ base down	$P_{H, \, sph} = 0.9^\Delta$ base in
$P_{V, \, cyl} = 0.92^\Delta$ base down	$P_{H, \, cyl} = 1.6^\Delta$ base in
Total $P_V = 2.12^\Delta$ base down	Total $P_H = 2.5^\Delta$ base in

Second method   *Prismatic effect due to the lens being considered as a crossed cylinder*

(i) Construct the vertical and horizontal meridians and the principal meridians of the lens; see figure 6.17. Using a convenient scale, locate the point D at which the prismatic effect is to be found. In this case, 4 mm above and 3 mm out from the optical centre.

Drop perpendiculars from D onto each principal meridian, meeting them at S and T.

Measure OS and OT. This procedure resolves the vertical and horizontal decentrations onto the principal meridians.

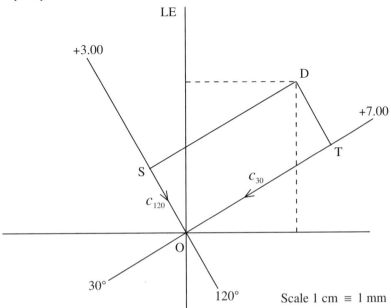

Fig. 6.17   **The horizontal, vertical, and principal meridians, and the decentrations for the second method in question 9.**

(ii) Measurement gives OS = 1.9 mm and OT = 4.6 mm. Now calculate the prismatic effects which will be produced along each principal meridian by the oblique decentrations OS and OT (c_{120} and c_{30}):

$$P_{120} = c_{120} \ |F_{120}| \ = 0.19 \times 3 \ = \ 0.57^\Delta \text{ base down } 120°.$$

This base direction is *down* because the power along this meridian is *plus*, and the optical centre O is *down* from the point S. That is, considering O to be 'decentred' down this meridian from the point D, the prism base is in the same direction as the decentration for a plus powered meridian.

$$P_{30} = c_{30} \ |F_{30}| \ = 0.46 \times 7 \ = \ 3.22^\Delta \text{ base down } 30°.$$

Similarly, the base direction is *down* 30° because the power along this meridian is *plus* and the optical O is *down* 30° from the point T.

(iii) Resolve these oblique prisms into their vertical and horizontal components; see figure 6.18.

Construct the vertical and horizontal meridians and the principal meridians. Using a convenient scale ($1'' \equiv 1^\Delta$) construct the prisms found in (ii) along each principal meridian in their stated base direction, and complete the rectangle OPRQ. Drop perpendiculars from R onto the vertical and horizontal meridians, meeting them at V and H, respectively. OV is the vertical prismatic effect and OH is the horizontal prismatic effect.

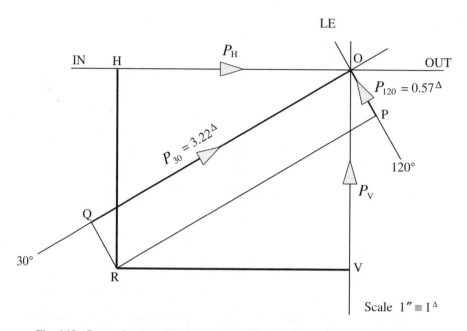

Fig. 6.18 Determination of the horizontal and vertical component prismatic effects.

By measurement from figure 6.18,

$$OV = P_V = 2.15^\Delta \text{ base down} \quad \text{and} \quad OH = P_H = 2.5^\Delta \text{ base in.}$$

---

10 Find the vertical and horizontal decentration required to produce the following prescription: R. −3.25 / −2.50 x 110 / 2$^\Delta$ base in / 1.5$^\Delta$ base up.

When a cylinder axis is oblique, a graphical method for obtaining the decentration may be found easier than an analytical method. In these cases, the lens should be considered as a crossed cylinder. The procedure is as follows:

(i) Resolve the prescribed prism into components along each principal meridian.

Method

Construct the vertical and horizontal meridians and the principal meridians of the lens. Using a convenient scale to represent the prisms, mark them off in their prescribed directions, OV = 1.5 and OH = 2.0, and complete the rectangle OVRH to obtain the resultant OR (P_R). See figure 6.19.

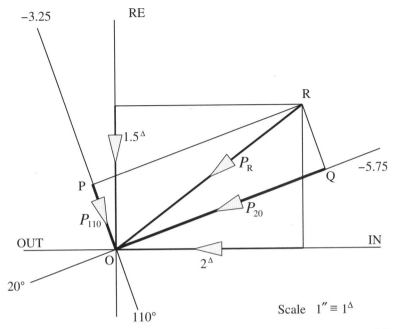

Fig. 6.19 The resultant prism P_R resolved into component prisms P_{20} and P_{110}.

Drop perpendiculars RP and RQ onto each principal meridian. The lengths OP and OQ represent the prisms (P_{110} and P_{20}) resolved onto each principal meridian. By measurement from figure 6.19, OP = P_{110} = 0.7$^\Delta$ base up 110° and OQ = 2.4$^\Delta$ base up 20°.

(ii) Using Prentice's Rule, calculate the decentration required to produce each of the prisms found in (i).

$$c_{110} = \frac{P_{110}}{|F_{110}|} = \frac{0.7}{3.25} = 0.22 \text{ cm} = 2.2 \text{ mm down } 110°$$

$$c_{20} = \frac{P_{20}}{|F_{20}|} = \frac{2.4}{5.75} = 0.42 \text{ cm} = 4.2 \text{ mm down } 20°.$$

Note: the rules governing the direction of the decentration were met in question 6.3. Here they are again for convenience:

*If the lens (or meridian) is **positive**, decentre in the **same** direction as the prism base.*
*If the lens (or meridian) is **negative**, decentre in the **opposite** direction to the prism base.*

(iii) Express the decentrations found in (ii) as vertical and horizontal components.

Method
Construct the vertical and horizontal meridians and the principal meridians of the lens. Scale-up the decentrations to a convenient size (1 cm ≡ 1 mm), and mark them off along the

67

principal meridians in the directions stated; see figure 6.20.

$$OS = c_{20} = 4.2 \text{ mm down } 20° \quad \text{and} \quad OT = c_{110} = 2.2 \text{ mm down } 110°.$$

Complete the rectangle OSDT. Note: if required, the single resultant decentration would be given be OD.

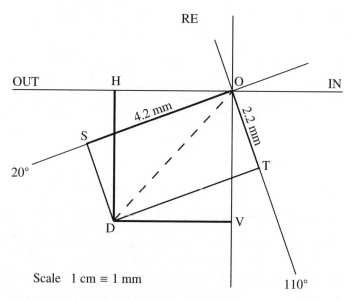

Scale 1 cm ≡ 1 mm

Fig. 6.20 **Obtaining the horizontal and vertical decentration components from the components along the principal meridians.**

To obtain the vertical and horizontal component decentrations, drop perpendiculars DV and DH. By measurement from figure 6.20,

$$OV = c_V = 3.5 \text{ mm down} \quad \text{and} \quad OH = c_H = 3.2 \text{ mm out.}$$

---

11 **At what point on the lens L. +3.75 / +2.50 x 55 will the wearer encounter 2^Δ base up and 0.5^Δ base out? Express your answer in vertical and horizontal terms.**

The construction is shown in question 6.10, except that the rules governing the direction of decentration do not apply in this case. Instead, the position of the point relative to the optical centre is obtained by inspection.

Method

(i) Resolve the prisms in the question into components along each principal meridian.
Construct the vertical and horizontal meridians and the principal meridians of the lens.

68

Using a convenient scale ($1'' \equiv 1^\Delta$) to represent the prisms, mark them off in their stated directions; see figure 6.21. $OV = 2$ and $OH = 0.5$. Note the scale; a rule with inches graduated in tenths is very useful. The other edge of the rule usually has centimetres for use with a scale 1 cm $\equiv$ 1 mm for decentration problems.

Complete the rectangle OVRH to obtain the resultant OR.

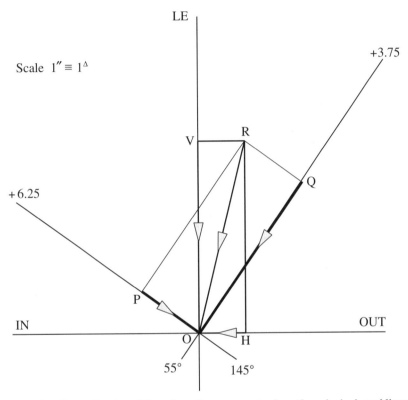

Fig. 6.21 Determination of the prismatic components along the principal meridians.

Drop perpendiculars RP and RQ onto each principal meridian. The lengths OP and OQ represent the prisms resolved onto each principal meridian.

$$OP = 0.75^\Delta \text{ base up } 145° \quad \text{and} \quad OQ = 1.92^\Delta \text{ base up } 55°.$$

(ii) Determine the distance from the visual point to the optical centre by using Prentice's Rule applied to each prism found in (i).

The direction along the principal meridians in which each point lies in relation to the optical centre is obtained by inspection. Thus, to obtain the base direction of the prism OP, the visual point must lie down and out from the optical centre since this is a positive meridian. Similarly, with the prism OQ, the visual point must lie down and in from the optical centre,

69

for the same reason. Hence,

$$c_{145} = \frac{P_{145}}{|F_{145}|} = \frac{0.75}{6.25} = 0.12 \text{ cm} = 1.2 \text{ mm down } 145°$$

and $\quad c_{55} = \frac{P_{55}}{|F_{55}|} = \frac{1.92}{3.75} = 0.51 \text{ cm} = 5.1 \text{ mm down } 55°.$

(iii) These oblique amounts must now be compounded to obtain a resultant which can then be expressed as vertical and horizontal components.

Method

Construct the vertical and horizontal meridians and the principal meridians of the lens. Scale-up the amounts to be compounded to a convenient size (1 cm $\equiv$ 1 mm), and mark them off along their respective meridians in the directions stated in (ii); see figure 6.22.

From part (ii), we have $\quad$ OS = 1.2 mm down 145° $\quad$ and $\quad$ OT = 5.1 mm down 55°. Complete the rectangle OSDT in figure 6.22.

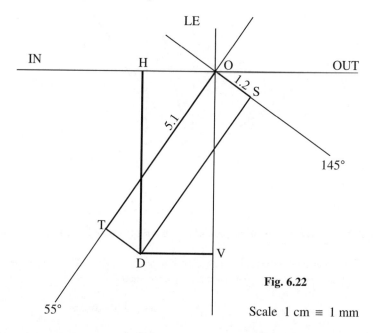

Fig. 6.22

Scale 1 cm $\equiv$ 1 mm

Although not shown in figure 6.22, OD is the resultant decentration. Now resolve the resultant into its horizontal and vertical components by dropping perpendiculars onto the horizontal and vertical meridians. That is, construct DH and DV.

By measurement, $\quad$ OH = 1.95 mm $\quad$ and $\quad$ OV = 4.9 mm.

Hence, the point D lies 4.9 mm below and 1.95 mm in from the optical centre of the lens.

12 A subject wearing the following prescription looks through points 5 mm below and 3 mm in from the optical centre of each lens. What horizontal and vertical differential prismatic effects would he encounter?

R.   +2.00 / +1.00 x 90   L. −1.00 / −2.00 x 180.

Explain how the term *differential prism* comes about.

Firstly, calculate the individual prismatic effects encountered by each eye.

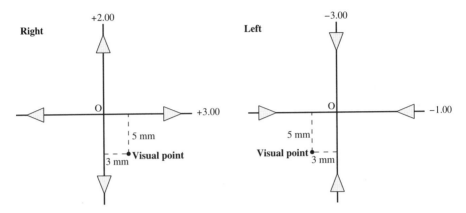

Fig. 6.23   The base directions of the horizontal and vertical prismatic effects at each visual point can be seen by inspection of these schematic diagrams.

Right

$P_V = c_V |F_V|$
$= 0.5 \times 2$
$= 1^\triangle$ base up

$P_H = c_H |F_H|$
$= 0.3 \times 3$
$= 0.9^\triangle$ base out

Left

$P_V = c_V |F_V|$
$= 0.5 \times 3$
$= 1.5^\triangle$ base down.

$P_H = c_H |F_H|$
$= 0.3 \times 1$
$= 0.3^\triangle$ base in.

To obtain the differential prism we must compare the prismatic effect in the right eye with the prismatic effect in the left eye. A simple rule is as follows:

If the base directions oppose each other, the prisms should be added.
If the bases are in the same direction, subtract the smaller prism from the larger.

Thus, considering the vertical prismatic effects above, we have:

$1^\triangle$ base up right and $1.5^\triangle$ base down left.

The bases are opposite, therefore we add the prisms, giving

$2.5^\triangle$ base up right, or $2.5^\triangle$ base down left.

Horizontally we have 0.9$^\Delta$ base out right and 0.3$^\Delta$ base in left.

The bases are in the same direction, therefore we subtract the smaller from the larger, giving

0.6$^\Delta$ base out right or 0.6$^\Delta$ base out left.

Alternative determination of the differential prismatic effects

The vertical prismatic effects are modelled with vector arrows in figure 6.24.

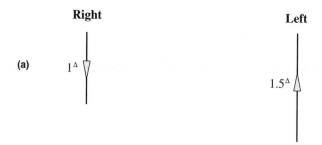

(a) The vertical prismatic effects at the visual points of the right and left lenses.

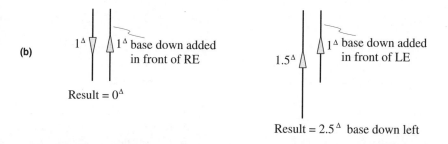

(b) The same 1$^\Delta$ base down prism is added in front of each eye. This is chosen to neutralise the prismatic effect in the right eye. The effect of adding 1$^\Delta$ base down in front of each eye is to make both eyes turn upwards through 1$^\Delta$, thus leaving the same angle between the visual axes, but now only the left eye is deviated and the differential (or relative) prismatic effect is obvious as 2.5$^\Delta$ base down left, the result shown above right.

Fig. 6.24 (a) and (b)   Determination of differential prism using vectors.

Repeating the exercise by adding 1.5$^\Delta$ base up before each eye makes the left prismatic effect go to zero and produces a differential prismatic effect of 2.5$^\Delta$ base up right.

The same method can be used for horizontal prismatic effects. Again, using the values for the prismatic effects obtained earlier: 0.9^Δ base out right and 0.3^Δ base in left.

Right   **Left**

(c)

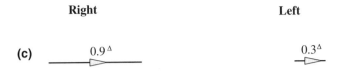

(c) The horizontal prismatic effects at the visual points of the right and left lenses.

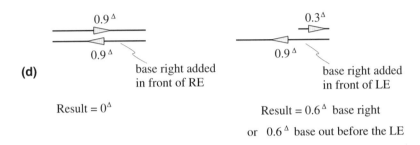

(d)   base right added   base right added
                          in front of RE   in front of LE

Result = 0^Δ Result = 0.6^Δ base right

                                        or 0.6^Δ base out before the LE

(d) The same 0.9^Δ base right prism is added in front of each eye. This is chosen to neutralise the prismatic effect in the right eye. The effect of adding 0.9^Δ base right in front of each eye is to make both eyes turn to the left through 0.9^Δ, thus leaving the same angle between prismatic effect is obvious as 0.6^Δ base out LE.
the visual axes, but now only the left eye is deviated and the differential (or relative)

Fig. 6.24(c) and (d) Determination of the horizontal differential prism using vectors.

One could do a head-to-tail addition of the prisms in front of the left eye to show the resultant is 0.6^Δ base out left eye, but above diagram should be sufficient to grasp the idea. Again, if the 0.3^Δ base left were added to each eye, the differential prism would come out as 0.6^Δ base left in front of the right eye (or 0.6^Δ base out right eye, in clinical notation).

The derivation of the term *differential prism*

In the example above, suppose base UP prism is given a PLUS sign and base DOWN a MINUS sign. Then, instead of R. 1^Δ base up and L. 1.5^Δ base down, we can write

R. $+1^\Delta$ and   L. -1.5^Δ.

The word *differential* means the result of subtracting two quantities. Suppose we subtract -1.5^Δ from the prisms in front of each eye, so that the angle between the two visual axes remains the same, then we have R. $(+1^\Delta) - (-1.5^\Delta) = +2.5^\Delta$ and L. $(-1.5^\Delta) - (-1.5^\Delta) = 0$.

73

That is, we have $+2.5^\Delta$ in front of the right eye, or 2.5^Δ base up in front of the right eye, and zero prism in front of the left eye. This is the result obtained earlier when using vectors and we see that we have obtained a *differential prism*. Because the prism in front of the left eye is zero, differential prism is sometimes called *relative prism*. That is, relative to the left eye the right eye here experiences 2.5^Δ base up.

---

13 A prescription reads **R. +1.75 / –3.00 x 90   L. +0.50 / –3.00 x 150. The lenses are correctly centred for distance. Calculate the prismatic effect of each lens at a point 8 mm below and 2 mm in from the optical centre. What are the vertical and horizontal differential prismatic effects?**

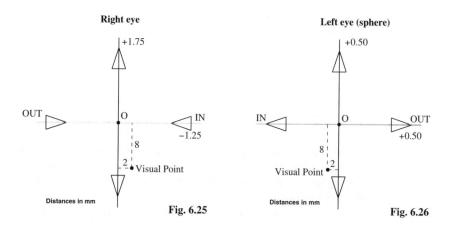

Right eye

Left eye (sphere)

Fig. 6.25

Fig. 6.26

Right Eye

The vertical and horizontal prismatic effects are calculated using figure 6.25.

$$P_V = c_V \, |F_V| = 0.8 \times 1.75 = 1.4^\Delta \text{ base up}$$

$$P_H = c_H \, |F_H| = 0.2 \times 1.25 = 0.25^\Delta \text{ base in}$$

Left eye

Using the graphical method as shown in question 6.8, calculate the prismatic effect due to the sphere and the cylinder separately; see figure 6.26 for the sphere.
(i) Prismatic effect due to the sphere:

$$P_V = c_V \, |F_V| = 0.8 \times 0.5 = 0.4^\Delta \text{ base up.}$$

$$P_H = c_H \, |F_H| = 0.2 \times 0.5 = 0.1^\Delta \text{ base out.}$$

74

(ii) Prismatic effect due to the cylinder in the left lens; see figure 6.27.

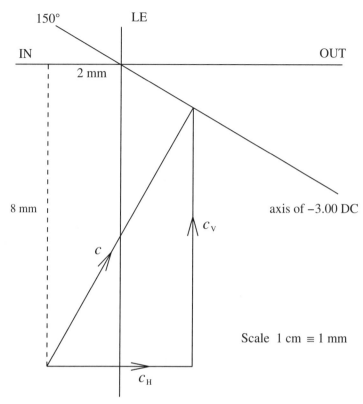

Fig. 6.27 The components c_V and c_H for the cylinder in the left lens.

By measurement, $c_V = 7$ mm and $c_H = 4$ mm.
This gives vertical and horizontal prismatic components of

$$P_V = c_V |F_V| = 0.7 \times 3 = 2.1^\Delta \text{ base down}$$

$$P_H = c_H |F_H| = 0.4 \times 3 = 1.2^\Delta \text{ base in.}$$

Adding together the prismatic effects of the sphere and the cylinder:

P_V due to the sphere $= 0.4^\Delta$ base up
P_V due to the cylinder $= 2.1^\Delta$ base down

Total $P_V = 1.7^\Delta$ base down.

P_H due to the sphere $= 0.1^\Delta$ base out
P_H due to the cylinder $= 1.2^\Delta$ base in

Total $P_H = 1.1^\Delta$ base in.

The differential prismatic effects are obtained by comparing those prismatic effects in the RE with those in the LE.

Vertical differential prismatic effect

The vertical prismatic effect in the right eye is 1.4^Δ base up, and in the left eye it is 1.7^Δ base down. The difference between them is $1.4 + 1.7 = 3.1^\Delta$ base up right, or base down left.

Alternatively, using the sign convention and subtracting the left prismatic effect from each eye gives $(+1.4^\Delta) - (-1.7^\Delta) = +3.1^\Delta$ in the right eye and $(-1.7^\Delta) - (-1.7^\Delta) = 0^\Delta$ in the left eye. That is, the differential prism is $+3.1^\Delta$ in the right eye, or 3.1^Δ base up in the right eye.

To see how this comes about we can look at the effect on the right and left visual axes. If the eyes are fixating a distant object point, the right eye will rotate downwards through an angle of 1.4^Δ whilst the left eye will rotate upwards through 1.7^Δ. The angle between the visual axes is 3.1^Δ. This angle could equally well be obtained by placing 3.1^Δ in front of one eye and no prism in front of the other.

Horizontal differential prismatic effect

The horizontal prismatic effect in the right eye is 0.25^Δ base in, and in the left eye it is 1.1^Δ base in. That is, the difference between them is $0.25 + 1.1 = 1.35^\Delta$ base in right or left.

Base in prism causes the visual axis to turn temporalwards. That is, the eye abducts. Since base in prism is before both eyes, they both abduct, resulting in an angle of 1.35^Δ between the visual axes when observing a distant point object. This could be achieved by making either the right or left eye abduct alone. 1.35^Δ base in before either the right or left eye would do this.

Again, the differential prismatic effect could be obtained using the sign convention applied to the prism base directions. Base in for the right eye is base to the right (+), and base in for the left eye is base to the left (−). Hence, making the prismatic effect in the left eye go to zero

gives   R. $(+0.25^\Delta) - (-1.1^\Delta) = +1.35^\Delta$ and   L. $(-1.1^\Delta) - (-1.1^\Delta) = 0^\Delta$, leaving 1.35^Δ base right or base in before the RE.

Problems solved using vector triangles

The preceding problems used mainly graphical constructions to solve them. This is a common method, but some students might prefer to use vector triangle solutions which lend themselves to simple trigonometrical calculations because the triangles are always right angled (since the principal meridians are orthogonal).

All problems involving prismatic effects or decentration reduce to the application of Prentice's Rule, either in the form giving prismatic effect when the decentration is known, or in the form giving decentration when the prismatic effect is known. That is,

$$P = c\,|F| \qquad \text{or} \qquad c = \frac{P}{|F|}\,.$$

We are either given c, directly or by implication, and we use the first form of Prentice's Rule above, or we are given P, as a single prism or as components, and we use the second form. That's really all there is to these problems.

If we are given the prismatic effect P, then we find its components along the two principal meridians and apply $c = P/|F|$ in each meridian to find the component decentrations in these meridians. Alternatively, if we are given the decentration c, we find its components in each principal meridian, apply $P = c\,|F|$, and find the component prismatic effect in each principal meridian. Once we have the required components of either the decentration or the prismatic effect, we can compound them to obtain the single resultant which may then be resolved into horizontal and vertical components if desired.

The method is best seen by example, and several problems are presented below. There are four types of problem which may be stated, but they reduce to only the two types of application of Prentice's Rule stated above. They are:

(1) *Given a decentration, find the prismatic effect it produces.*
(2) *Find the prismatic effect at a point on a lens.*
(3) *Given a prismatic effect, find the decentration which produces it.*
(4) *Find the point on a lens at which a given prismatic effect is present.*

Problem type (2) can be re-expressed as problem type (1), and problem type (4) can be re-expressed as type (3), leaving us with just two problem types which each depend on one form of Prentice's Rule as stated above.

14 **Problem Type (1). A lens with the prescription L. –2.00 / –4.00 x 20 is decentred 6 mm up 150°. Calculate the single resultant prismatic effect and express it in its horizontal and vertical components.**

We are given the decentration c so, in order to use Prentice's Rule, we must find its components c_{20} and c_{110} along the principal meridians. This we do in figure 6.28 which has been drawn to scale.

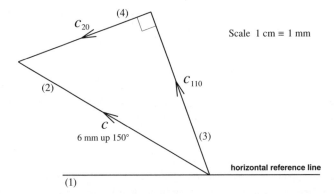

Scale 1 cm ≡ 1 mm

Fig. 6.28   **The diagram shows the given decentration c = 6 mm up 150°, constructed using a protractor and a ruler. These diagrams always commence with a horizontal reference line and the number (1) adjacent to this line indicates it was drawn first. The other numbers indicate the order in which they were constructed, using a ruler, a protractor for the angle 110° and the direction of c_{110}, and a set-square to construct the right angle and c_{20}. The component decentrations could easily be calculated, but since the figure is drawn to scale it is sufficiently accurate to measure them. Note that the arrows on the components indicate the vectors lead from the start of the single decentration c to its end. This is *vector addition*.**

By measurement from the diagram, c_{20} = 3.9 mm down 20° and c_{110} = 4.6 mm up 110°.

Using Prentice's Rule, the prismatic effects produced by these component decentrations are

$$P_{20} = c_{20} \, |F_{20}| = 0.39 \times 2 = 0.78^{\triangle} \text{ base up } 20°$$

and $$P_{110} = c_{110} \, |F_{110}| = 0.46 \times 6 = 2.76^{\triangle} \text{ base down } 110°.$$

Note: the rules governing the determination of the prism base direction are:

*If the meridian has **plus power**, the prism base is in the **same** direction as the decentration.*
*If the meridian has **minus power**, the prism base is in the **opposite** direction to the decentration.*

The single resultant prismatic effect is found by compounding (adding vectorially) the two component prismatic effects just found (P_{20} = 0.78△ base up 20° and P_{110} = 2.76△ base down 110°), as shown in figure 6.29.

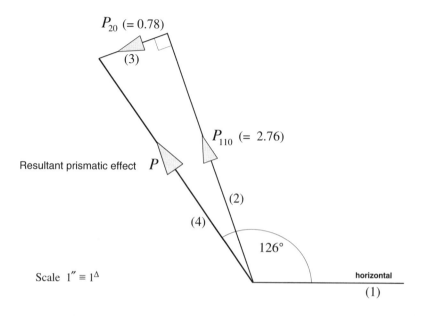

Fig. 6.29   **Construction of the vector triangle to determine the single resultant prismatic effect from the component prismatic effects P_{20} and P_{110} calculated earlier. The numbers in brackets again indicate the order in which the diagram was drawn.**

By measurement in figure 6.29, the single resultant prismatic effect is $P = 2.9$△ and the angle P makes with the horizontal is 126°. To obtain the prism base direction, note that P_{110} and P_{20} must run 'head-to-tail' from the starting point on the horizontal reference line to the finishing point which is at the upper left hand of the diagram. The resultant P must also 'run' from the starting point to the same finishing point, so the prism arrow must be as shown. The arrow is then regarded as a prism in order to describe its base direction. Evidently, by measurement from the diagram, the resultant is $P = 2.85$△ down 126°.

The horizontal and vertical components of the resultant prismatic effect P are determined from figure 6.30. By measurement from the scale diagram, the horizontal component is $P_H = 1.7$△ base out (by inspection of the vector construction). The vertical component is $P_V = 2.3$△ base down.

79

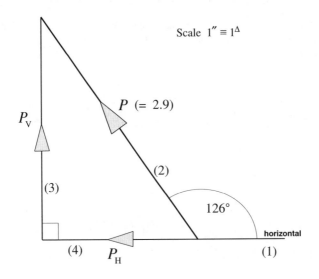

Scale $1'' \equiv 1^\Delta$

Fig. 6.30   Determination of the horizontal and vertical components (P_H and P_V).
Again, the numbers indicate the order in which the diagram was
constructed, and the prism arrows follow the rules of vector addition.

---

15   **Type 2 problem. A lens has the prescription R. +3.50 / –1.50 x 120. Find the prismatic
effect at the point 4 mm out and 7 mm down from the optical centre O.**

This type of question can be thought of in a way which changes it into a type 1 question; that
is, a question where we have a decentration and we are asked to find the consequent
prismatic effect. Refer to figure 6.31. The legend explains the principle of converting this
type of question into one where we think in decentration terms — its simply a ruse which
some of us find convenient. The figure shows the horizontal and vertical meridians, and the
axis meridian 120°. RM is perpendicular to the axis meridian and therefore lies along the
30° meridian. Hence, we can find the decentrations c_{30} and c_{120} along the 30° and 120°
meridians from the diagram, which is drawn to the scale 1 cm $\equiv$ 1 mm.

By measurement, $c_{30} = RM = 6.9$ mm up 30°   and $c_{120} = MO = 4.1$ mm up 120°.   Hence,
we can find the prismatic effects along these meridians:

First, $P_{30} = c_{30}\,|F_{30}| = 0.69 \times 2.00 = 1.38^\Delta$ base up 30°.

Note that the principal powers are +2.00 D along 30° and +3.50 along 120°, and decentration
in a given direction along a positive powered meridian produces a prismatic effect with its
base in the *same* direction.

Then, $P_{120} = c_{120}\,|F_{120}| = 0.41 \times 3.50 = 1.44^\Delta$ base up 120°.

Right lens

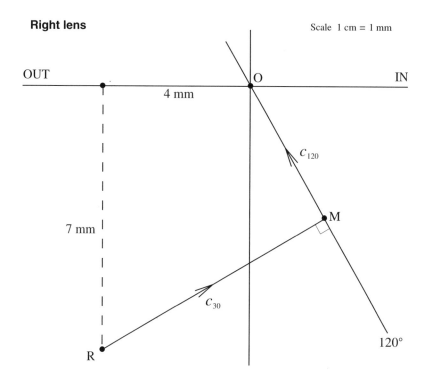

Fig. 6.31   The exercise is to find the prismatic effect at the point R, a distance 4 mm out and 7 mm down from the optical centre O. However, we think of this as a decentration statement where, along the principal meridians, the optical centre O is considered to be decentred c_{30} followed by c_{120} from the point R. We then use these decentrations to calculate the prismatic effect components P_{30} and P_{120}.

The single resultant prismatic effect is found by adding these component prismatic effects vectorially, as in figure 6.32. Note, again, that when forming the vector triangle the components P_{30} and P_{120} are placed with their 'arrows' head-to-tail. The resultant P must be directed from the same starting point to the same finishing point to complete the triangle.

Fig. 6.32

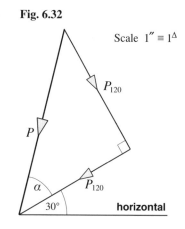

By measurement from figure 6.32, we have $P = 2.0^{\Delta}$ base up $\alpha + 30°$. and $\alpha = 46°$, so we have $P = 2.0^{\Delta}$ base up $76°$.

It might be considered that finding c_{30} and c_{120} by measurement from figure 6.31 is simpler than using trigonometry, but since figure 6.32 is a simple right-angled triangle the trigonometrical solution for P is comparatively simple. Thus, since $P_{30} = 1.38^\Delta$ and $P_{120} = 1.44^\Delta$, by Pythagoras' Theorem,

$$P = \sqrt{P_{30}^2 + P_{120}^2} = \sqrt{1.38^2 + 1.44^2} = 1.99^\Delta.$$

Then, for α, $\tan \alpha = \dfrac{P_{120}}{P_{30}} = \dfrac{1.44}{1.38} = 1.04$

from which $\alpha = 46.1°$.

Suppose we were asked for the horizontal and vertical components of the single resultant prism P, then the procedure is identical to that used in figure 6.30 in the previous problem. One could simplify the procedure by drawing P_H and P_V on the diagram used to determine P, that is, on figure 6.32. It makes it look a little more complex, but if done in a different colour the detail stands out sufficiently. Figure 6.33(a) illustrates this idea, and figure 6.33(b) shows the construction of P, P_H and P_V alone, for those who would prefer to keep each stage on a separate diagram.

Fig. 6.33

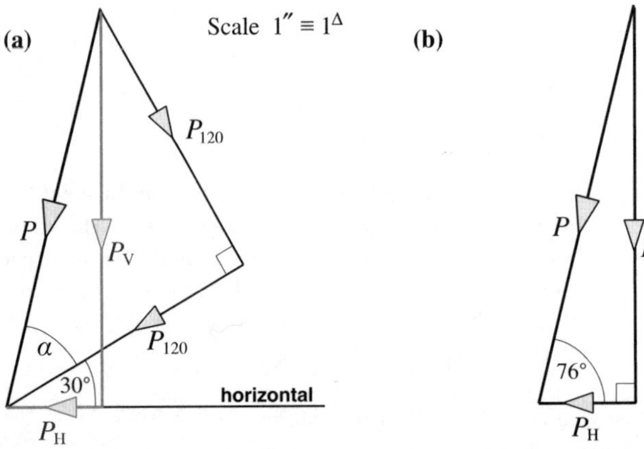

By calculation,

$$P_H = P \cos 76° = 1.99 \times 0.2419 = 0.48^\Delta \text{ base in (its a right lens)}$$

and $P_V = P \sin 76° = 1.99 \times 0.9703 = 1.93^\Delta \text{ base up.}$

with the base direction taken from the diagram. Measurement from the diagram gives closely similar results ($P_H = 0.49^\Delta$ and $P_V = 1.9^\Delta$).

16 **A type 3 problem. For the lens R. –3.00 / –2.00 x 70, (i) find the single decentration which will produce 1ᐃ base in and 2ᐃ base down, (ii) determine the horizontal and vertical components of this decentration.**

First find the single prismatic effect (P) by vector addition of P_H and P_V, the stated horizontal and vertical prisms. When we have P we then find P_{70} and P_{160}, the components of P in the principal meridians. These components will then allow us to find the component decentrations c_{70} and c_{160}.

The single prismatic effect P is determined with the aid of figure 6.34(a) below.

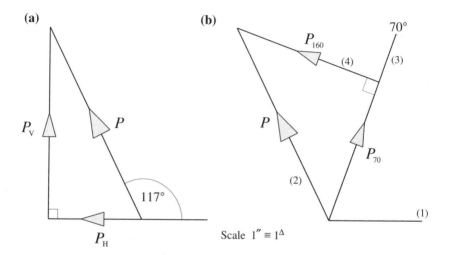

Fig. 6.34 (a) Vector triangle used to determine the single prismatic effect (P) by vector addition of the given prism components P_H and P_V.

(b) Determination of the prism components along the 70° and 160° meridians. The numbers on the various lines indicate the order in which they were drawn.

By measurement, from figure 6.34(a), $P = 2.2^\Delta$ along 117°. The base is seen to be down 117° from the vector triangle construction. Using figure 6.34(b), constructed in the order indicated by the numbers in brackets, the component prisms along the 70° and 160° meridians are, by measurement, $P_{70} = 1.5^\Delta$ base down 70° and $P_{160} = 1.6^\Delta$ base down 160°.

We may now calculate the decentrations along the 70° and 160° meridians:

$$c_{70} = \frac{P_{70}}{|F_{70}|} = \frac{1.5}{3} = 0.5 \text{ cm} = 5 \text{ mm up } 70°.$$

The decentration is *up* 70° since the prismatic effect is *base down* on a negative meridian power (–3.00 D).

83

Next, $c_{160} = \dfrac{P_{160}}{|F_{160}|} = \dfrac{1.6}{5} = 0.32\,\text{cm} = 3.2\,\text{mm up }160°$

since the power along 160° is –5.00 D. The single decentration is now found by vector addition of the components c_{70} and c_{160}, as shown in figure 6.35.

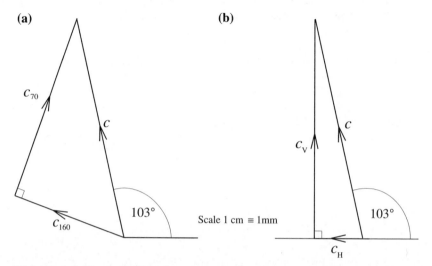

(a) c_{70} c 103° c_{160}

Scale 1 cm ≡ 1mm

(b) c c_V 103° c_H

Fig. 6.35 (a)   **Vector addition of component decentrations c_{70} and c_{160} to determine the single resultant decentration c.**
       (b)   **Determination of the horizontal and vertical components of c.**

By measurement from figure 6.35(a), the resultant decentration is $c = 5.9$ mm up 103°. From part (b) of this figure, $c_H = 1.3$ mm out and $c_V = 5.7$ mm up.

Although much of the above data have been taken from scale diagrams, one should be able to appreciate how easy trigonometry can be applied to these figures.

THE NEXT THREE QUESTIONS USE FORMULAE METHODS

17 Use Cartesian sign convention formulae to calculate the horizontal and vertical prismatic effects at the point 7 mm below and 3 mm in from the optical centre of the lens R. −2.50 / −3.25 x 70. (Note that this is question 8 again!)

The equations required are: $\qquad H = -xF_s + \{y\cos\theta - x\sin\theta\}\,F_c\sin\theta$

and $\qquad V = -yF_s - \{y\cos\theta - x\sin\theta\}\,F_c\cos\theta$

where H and V are the horizontal and vertical prismatic effects at the point (x, y) on the lens, measured from the optical centre as origin. x is positive when the point is to the right of the optical centre O, and negative when it is to the left of O. y is positive when the point is above O and negative when it is below O. x and y should be entered in centimetres since the equations are derived using Prentice's Rule.

F_s and F_c are the sphere and cyl powers, and θ is the cyl axis.

Hence, $\quad H = -xF_s + \{y\cos\theta - x\sin\theta\}\,F_c\sin\theta$
$$= -(+0.3)\times(-2.50) + \{(-0.7)\cos 70° - (+0.3)\sin 70°\}\times(-3.25)\sin 70°$$
$$= +0.75 + \{(-0.2394) - (+0.2819)\}\times(-3.0540)$$
$$= +0.75 + 1.5920$$
$$= +2.342\,^\triangle$$
the plus sign indicating the base is to the right, which is base in on a right lens.

Next, $\quad V = -yF_s - \{y\cos\theta - x\sin\theta\}\,F_c\cos\theta$
$$= -(-0.7)\times(-2.50) + \{(-0.7)\cos 70° - (+0.3)\sin 70°\}\times(-3.25)\cos 70°$$
$$= -1.75 - \{(-0.2394) - (+0.2819)\}\times(-1.1116)$$
$$= -1.75 - (+0.5795)$$
$$= -2.330\,^\triangle, \text{ or } 2.330\,^\triangle \text{ base down,}$$

the minus sign indicating base down in the sign convention used.

In modern practice, such analytical techniques are used in computer programs. Graphical techniques undertaken by students are valuable in so far as they give the student a feel for the effects of decentration and prism.

---

18 On the lens R. −3.25 / −2.50 x 110, use Cartesian sign convention equations to find the horizontal and vertical decentrations required to produce $2^\triangle$ base in and $1.5^\triangle$ base up . (Note that this is question 10 again.)

The equations required are $\quad c_H = \dfrac{\{F_s + F_c\cos^2\theta\}\,H + \{F_c\sin\theta\cos\theta)\,V}{F_s(F_s + F_c)}$

and $\quad c_V = \dfrac{\{F_c\sin\theta\cos\theta\}\,H + \{F_s + F_c\sin^2\theta)\,V}{F_s(F_s + F_c)}$.

The distances c_H and c_V are the horizontal and vertical decentrations. The other symbols are the same as in question 17. Decentration up is positive, down negative, right positive, and left negative.

Hence, the horizontal decentration is

$$c_H = \frac{\{F_s + F_c \cos^2 \theta\}\, H \; + \; \{F_c \sin \theta \cos \theta)\, V}{F_s(F_s + F_c)}$$

$$= \frac{\{(-3.25) + (-2.50) \cos^2 110°\} \times (+2) \; + \; \{(-2.50) \sin 110° \cos 110°\} \times (+1.5)}{(-3.25) \times \{(-3.25) + (-2.50)\}}$$

$$= -0.3146 \text{ cm}$$

$$= -3.146 \text{ mm}.$$

The negative sign indicates a decentration to the left, which is *out* for a right eye.

The vertical decentration is

$$c_V = \frac{\{F_c \sin \theta \cos \theta\}\, H \; + \; \{F_s + F_c \sin^2 \theta\,)\, V}{F_s(F_s + F_c)} .$$

$$= \frac{\{(-2.50) \sin 110° \cos 110°\} \times (+2) \; + \; \{(-3.25) + (-2.50) \sin^2 110°\} \times (+1.5)}{(-3.25) \times \{(-3.25) + (-2.50)\}}$$

$$= -0.3521 \text{ cm}$$

$$= -3.521 \text{ mm}.$$

The negative sign indicates a decentration downwards.

---

19 Find the point on the lens +3.00 / −7.00 x 130 at which there is a prismatic effect $P = 2^\Delta$ base down 150°.

Figure 6.36 shows the single prism, from which its horizontal and vertical components are:

$H = P \cos 150° = (-2) \cos 150°$
$\quad = +1.732^\Delta$
and
$V = P \sin 150° = (-2) \sin 150°$
$\quad = -1.0^\Delta.$

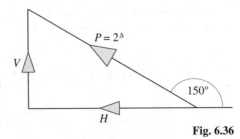

$P = 2^\Delta$

V

H

150°

Note that the external angle (standard notation) must be used, and that 'base down' at any angle to the horizontal is given a minus sign.

Fig. 6.36

Thus, $P = -2^{\Delta}$ along $150°$ means the same as 2^{Δ} base down $150°$.

The equations required are obtained from those in question 17, solved for x and y:

$$x = \frac{\{F_s + F_c \cos^2 \theta\}\, H \; + \; \{F_c \sin \theta \cos \theta)\, V}{- F_s(F_s + F_c)}$$

$$y = \frac{\{F_c \sin \theta \cos \theta\}\, H \; + \; \{F_s + F_c \sin^2 \theta)\, V}{- F_s(F_s + F_c)}.$$

The origin is at the optical centre, so x and y are relative to the optical centre as usual. Notice how these equations differ only from those in question 18 by a minus sign in the denominator. This indicates the reverse nature between finding the decentration to produce a given prismatic effect and finding the prismatic effect at a given point (problem types 3 and 4 on page 77).

Hence,

$$x = \frac{\{F_s + F_c \cos^2 \theta\}\, H \; + \; \{F_c \sin \theta \cos \theta)\, V}{- F_s(F_s + F_c)}$$

$$= \frac{\{(+3) + (-7)\cos^2 130°\} \times (+1.732) \; + \; (-7)\sin 130° \cos 130° \times (-1)}{-(+3) \times ((+3)+(-7))}$$

$$= -0.272 \text{ cm.}$$

and

$$y = \frac{\{F_c \sin \theta \cos \theta\}\, H \; + \; \{F_s + F_c \sin^2 \theta)\, V}{- F_s(F_s + F_c)}.$$

$$= \frac{(-7)\sin 130° \cos 130° \times (+1.732) \; + \; ((+3)+(-7)\sin^2 130°) \times (-1)}{-(+3) \times ((+3)+(-7))}$$

$$= +0.590 \text{ cm.}$$

That is, the point is 2.72 mm down and 5.90 mm to the right of the optical centre.

One word of warning: notice that the denominators of these equations go to zero in the case of a plano-cylinder, when $F_s = 0$. This is because there is no unique point on such a lens for a given prismatic effect. For example, a +1.00 DC with its axis at $180°$ will have 1^{Δ} base down at all points 1 cm above the horizontal meridian where the lens is thickest.

20 A plano-convex bicentric lens of power −6.25 D is flat-edged round and 42 mm in diameter. The optical centre of the distance portion is at the geometric centre of the lens, which is 5 mm above the dividing line. The thick edge substance is 4.5 mm and the thin edge substance is 2.9 mm. Calculate the position of the optical centre of the reading portion. $n = 1.525$.

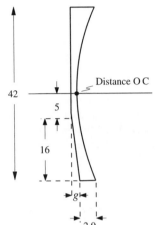

Fig. 6.37

The slabbed-off lens.
(Distances in mm.)

The amount of prism which has been slabbed-off can be calculated using the prism edge thickness difference formula,

$$g = \frac{Pd}{100\,(n-1)} \quad \text{rearranged to} \quad P = \frac{100\,(n-1)g}{d}.$$

In figure 6.37, $g = 4.5 - 2.9 = 1.6$ mm is the edge thickness difference of a prism whose aperture is $d = 16$ mm.

Hence, $\quad P = \dfrac{100\,(n-1)g}{d} = \dfrac{100 \times (1.525 - 1) \times 1.6}{16} = 5.25^{\Delta}.$

That is, 5.25^{Δ} base down has been removed, or, to put it another way, 5.25^{Δ} has been effectively added base up. The distance which the optical centre would have to move in order to create 5.25^{Δ} base up can be found using Prentice's Rule:

$$c = \frac{P}{|F|} = \frac{5.25}{6.25} = 0.84 \text{ cm} \quad \text{or} \quad 8.4 \text{ mm downwards.}$$

So, the optical centre of the reading portion is 8.4 mm below the distance optical centre.

Alternative solution

In figure 6.38, since the optical centre of a plano-concave lens lies on the back surface of the lens, O_D and O_N are the optical centres of the distance and near portions of the bi-centric lens. Let δ be the distance of O_N below the optical axis of the distance portion. $O_N C_2$ is the optical axis of the near portion and, from the diagram, it can be seen that this makes an angle α with the distance optical axis $O_D C_2$.

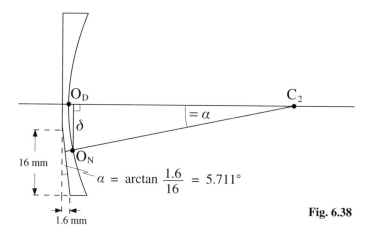

$$\alpha = \arctan \frac{1.6}{16} = 5.711°$$

Fig. 6.38

Hence, $\delta = O_N C_2 \times \sin \alpha = r_2 \sin \alpha = \dfrac{n_2' - n_2}{F_2} \times \sin \alpha$, where δ will be in metres.

For δ in mm, multiply by 1000, so

$$\delta = 1000 \times \frac{n_2' - n_2}{F_2} \times \sin \alpha = 1000 \times \frac{(1 - 1.525)}{-6.25} \times \sin 5.711° = 8.4 \text{ mm}.$$

7 MINIMUM SIZE OF UNCUT AND FIELD OF VIEW

1   A distance prescription reads

R. $-5.00 / -2.00 \times 180 / 3^\Delta$ base in   L. $-5.00 / -3.00 \times 180 / 3^\Delta$ base in.

The Boxed Centre Distance (boxed CD) of the frame is 70 mm and the lens size is 52 mm round. If the patient's PD is 66 mm, find the decentration required for each lens and the minimum size of uncut(MSU) that can be used if the prism is to be obtained by decentration.

Since the cyls contribute no power horizontally we only need to consider the spheres. The same calculation will suffice for both lenses since the spheres are both -5.00 D. In order to produce 3^Δ base in we must decentre each lens by a distance c given by

$$c = \frac{P}{|F|} = \frac{3}{5} = 0.6 \text{ cm} = 6 \text{ mm out.}$$

For distance vision, this 3^Δ prismatic effect must be placed in front of the pupil centre at what is known as the centration point (C) in the frame lens aperture, which is 2 mm IN from the boxed centre B, as determined below:

$$\frac{boxed\ CD - PD}{2} = \frac{70 - 66}{2} = 2 \text{ mm IN from the boxed centre.}$$

Therefore, in addition, the lens must be decentred IN by 2 mm to place the 3^Δ prismatic effect in front of the pupil centre, at C, when looking in the distance.

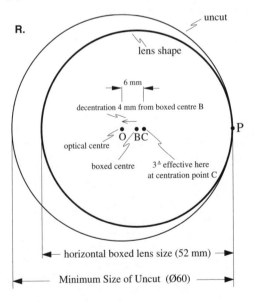

Fig. 7.1   Diagram drawn to actual size.

The resultant decentration is   6 mm out + 2 mm in = 4 mm out.

Figure 7.1 shows the lens size (bold circle), 52 mm in diameter and round in shape, with the boxed centre B and the optical centre (O) 4 mm out from B on this right lens. The uncut's radius must be OP, at least.
Now, OP = OB + BP = 4 + (½ × 52) = 30 mm.   So the $MSU = 2$ OP $= 2 \times 30 = 60$ mm.

Note that the minimum size uncut is also give by

$$MSU = horizontal\ boxed\ lens\ size + (2 \times decentration).$$

---

2   **Find the minimum size of uncut to produce the glazed lens L. –4.00 / –2.00 x 90 with 4^{Δ} base up 60° by decentration effective (i) at the boxed centre of a 44 mm round lens shape, and (ii) at a point 3 mm in from the boxed centre.**

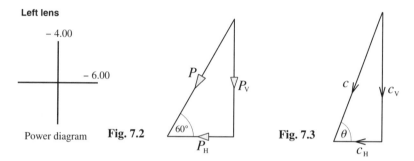

Left lens

Power diagram   **Fig. 7.2**   **Fig. 7.3**

(i)   We need to resolve the 4^{Δ} base up 60° into components along 180° and 90°, the directions of the principal meridians. From figure 7.2, the horizontal and vertical prism components are:

$$P_H = P \cos 60° = 4 \times 0.5 = 2^{\Delta}\ base\ out$$

and $$P_V = P \sin 60° = 4 \times 0.866 = 3.46^{\Delta}\ base\ up.$$

The corresponding horizontal and vertical decentrations are:

$$c_H = \frac{P_H}{|F_H|} = \frac{2}{6} = 0.33\ cm = 3.3\ mm\ IN.$$

(The decentration is IN to produce base OUT prism on a minus meridian.)

$$c_V = \frac{P_V}{|F_V|} = \frac{3.46}{4} = 0.87\ cm = 8.7\ mm\ DOWN.$$

The single resultant decentration, c, can be found from the vector triangle in figure 7.3.

Hence, $c = \sqrt{c_H^2 + c_V^2} = \sqrt{3.3^2 + 8.7^2} = 9.3$ mm down the θ meridian

where $\theta = \arctan \dfrac{8.7}{3.3} = 69.2°$.

Decentering the lens 9.3 mm down the 69.2° meridian from the boxed centre will produce the required prism. From the last question, since the lens shape is round the minimum size uncut is given by the *boxed lens size + twice the decentration*. For a round shape the boxed size is 44 □ 44, so we do not need to specify the horizontal measurement explicitly!

So, MSU = *boxed lens size* + $(2 \times decentration)$ = $44 + (2 \times 9.3)$ = 62.6 mm.

(ii) If the prism is to be effective at a point 3 mm in from the boxed centre, we must move the lens bodily 3 mm in from the position calculated in (i). That is, a further decentration in addition to the 9.3 mm down 69.2°. This is shown in figure 7.4, where the new resultant decentration is c_n (subscript n for new).

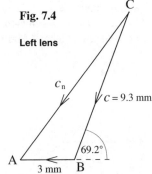

Fig. 7.4

Left lens

Figure 7.4 is not drawn to scale, so by calculation, using the cosine rule,

$c_n{}^2 = AB^2 + BC^2 - 2 AB \cdot BC \cos \angle ABC$

$\quad = 3^2 + 9.3^2 - 2 \times 3 \times 9.3 \cos 110.8°$

$\quad = 9 + 86.49 - (2 \times 3 \times 9.3 \times (-0.3551))$

$\quad = 115.3$.

So, c_n = $\sqrt{115.3}$ = 10.7 mm.

Thus, the minimum size uncut is

MSU = *boxed lens size* + $(2 \times decentration)$ = $44 + (2 \times 10.7)$ = 65.4 mm.

Using the sine rule to find the direction of decentration (c_n), the angle CAB,

$$\sin \angle CAB = 9.3 \times \frac{\sin \angle ABC}{c_n} = 9.3 \times \frac{\sin 110.8°}{10.7} = 0.8125 ,$$

whence $\angle CAB$ = $\arcsin 0.8125$ = $54.3°$.

---

4   **Figure 7.5 shows a lens shape with horizontal boxed lens size 58 mm. It is to be glazed with decentration BC = 5 mm in. Find the minimum size of uncut (MSU) required, and derive an approximate rule for finding the MSU. That is, derive the rule**
$MSU \approx$ horizontal boxed lens size $+$ (2 × decentration).

In figure 7.5, B is the boxed centre, C is the centration point where the optical centre will be placed in this case, and R is a point on the edge of the lens furthest from C. So, RC is the minimum radius of the uncut from which this lens can be glazed.

By measurement, the MSU will need a minimum diameter of $2\,RC$ = 2×35 = 70 mm.

From the triangle RBC, RC < (RB + BC), so 2 RC < 2 (RB + BC).

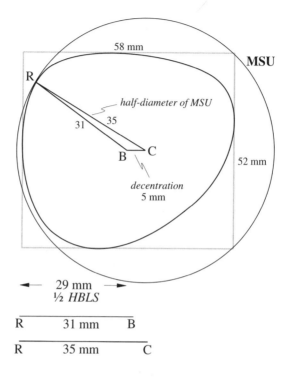

R	31 mm	B

R	35 mm	C

Fig. 7.5 **Full-size boxed lens shape. ½ *HBLS* is half the Horizontal Boxed Lens Size. Note that the longest semi-chord from the boxed centre B to the furthest edge (R) of the lens is such that RB ≈ ½ *HBLS*. This observation holds reasonably well for all lens shapes.**

Now, MSU = 2 RC

so MSU = 2 RC < 2 (RB + BC) = 2 RB + 2 BC = 2 RB + (2 × *decentration*).

But, 2 RB > *HBLS* (Horizontal Boxed Lens Size) of the frame.

So, *MSU* ≈ *HBLS* + (2 × *decentration*).

We have already determined the accurate MSU at 70 mm diameter, by measurement (2 RC) from the diagram. The approximation above gives

$$MSU \approx HBLS + (2 \times decentration) = 58 + (2 \times 5) = 68$$

giving an estimate of MSU 2 mm smaller than required. We see the rule is useful, as a guide, but not exact. In practice, a lens uncut size gauge would be used to determine the exact Minimum Size Uncut required. One should note that the Datum System is still used in workshop practice in the UK and the approximation in that case is

$$MSU \approx longest\ diameter\ across\ the\ lens\ shape\ +\ (\ 2 \times decentration)$$

the decentration being from the datum centre of the frame lens shape in this case.

---

5   A +10.00 D lens, 42 mm in diameter, is worn 25 mm from the centre of rotation of the eye. Find the fixation field of view. An axial point object, 1 m from the lens, is moved upwards and is seen to disappear. On moving further upwards it again becomes visible. Find the radial extent of the blind region (i.e. the width of the ring scotoma). Assume the lens is a rimless mount.

Figure 7.6 shows the lens, assumed thin, and the eye rotated through θ' to regard the object at B_1. After B_1 , until the object point reaches B_2 when it can be seen over the lens, the point cannot be imaged at the centre of the macula; that is, it cannot be fixated over the distance B_1B_2 . So, B_1B_2 is the radial extent of the ring scotoma.

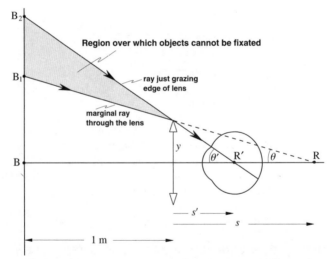

Fig. 7.6 B_1B_2 represents the width of the annulus over which the eye cannot fixate an object point. If the shaded area is rotated through 360° about the axis, it defines a region of space called a ring scotoma.

From the figure, $B_1B_2 = BB_2 - BB_1 = (1 + s') \tan \theta' - (1 + s) \tan \theta$ (1).

We must find s, $\tan \theta$, and $\tan \theta'$. s' is given as 25 mm ($= 0.025$ m).

Firstly, from the figure, $\tan \theta' = \dfrac{y}{s'} = \dfrac{21}{25}$ where $y = 21$ mm, half the lens diameter.

Next, $\tan \theta = \frac{y}{s}$. But we need s before we can find $\tan \theta$!

Assuming the thin lens equation is valid for angles as large a θ (which it really is not), we can find $\tan \theta$ as follows. Regarding R as a virtual object, then the object and image distances are s and s', respectively. R' is the centre of rotation of the eye. Then,

$$\frac{1}{s'} - \frac{1}{s} = \frac{1}{f'}, \quad \text{or} \quad \frac{1}{s} = \frac{1}{s'} - \frac{1}{f'} = \frac{1}{+25} - \frac{1}{+100} = \frac{3}{+100} \tag{2}$$

where $s' = +25$ mm and the focal length of the thin lens is $f' = +100$ mm.

Hence, $s = +33.3$ mm.

$$\text{So,} \quad \tan \theta = \frac{y}{s} = y \times \frac{1}{s} = 21 \times \frac{3}{100} = \frac{63}{100} \tag{3}.$$

From equation (2), $s = 33.3$ mm = 0.0333 m, so equation (1) can now be evaluated:

$$B_1B_2 = (1 + s') \tan \theta' - (1 + s) \tan \theta$$

$$= \left\{ (1 + 0.025) \times \frac{21}{25} \right\} - \left\{ (1 + 0.0333) \times \frac{63}{100} \right\}$$

$$= 0.861 - 0.651$$

$$= 0.21 \text{ m}.$$

That is, the radial extent of the ring scotoma is 21 cm. The object space fixation field of view is θ, in angular terms, or BB_1 in linear terms, where

$$BB_1 = BR \tan \theta = 1.0333 \times \frac{63}{100} = 0.6510 \text{ m} = 651 \text{ mm}.$$

In image space, the fixation field of view is the ocular rotation θ'.

$$\theta' = \arctan \frac{21}{25} = 40°, \text{ which is close to the eye's maximum of about } 50°.$$

8 BIFOCALS AND TRIFOCALS

1 The prescription −8.00 / +2.00 x 90, Add +2.50, is made as a round segment fused bifocal in glasses of refractive indices 1.52 and 1.65 for the main lens and the segment, respectively. The segment is on the spherical surface. If it is made on (a) a −10.00 D base curve (b) a +2.00 D base curve, find the power of the depression curve in each case.

Part (a) From first principles, and assuming the lens is thin, we have

$$Addition = Reading\ portion\ power - Distance\ portion\ power \qquad (1).$$

Using the following symbols which, except for A, will be found in figure 8.1(a),

A = Addition
F_1 = power of front surface in the distance portion
F_2 = power of back surface in the distance and near portions
$F_{1,s}$ = power of the front surface over the segment
F_{con} = power of the contact surface between the segment button and the main lens.

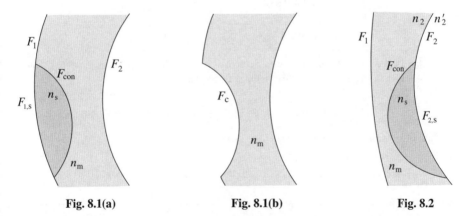

| Fig. 8.1(a) | Fig. 8.1(b) | Fig. 8.2 |

Since, for a thin lens, the power is the sum of the surface powers, equation (1) becomes

$$A = (F_{1,s} + F_{con} + F_2) - (F_1 + F_2) = F_{1,s} + F_{con} - F_1$$

which rearranges to give $\qquad F_{con} = A + F_1 - F_{1,s}$ \qquad (2).

Once we have the power (F_{con}) of the contact surface, it is a simple matter to find its radius. We now need to find the values of the terms F_1 and $F_{1,s}$ on the right hand side of equation (2). The lens is made on a −10.00 D base curve, so the distance portion has a thin lens toric transposition of

$$\frac{+4.00\ DS}{-10.00\ DC\ x\ 90\ /\ -12.00\ DC\ x\ 180}\ .$$

From this written transposition, the front surface power in the distance portion is $F_1 = +4.00$ D. The power $F_{1,s}$ of the front surface of the segment is found as follows, with $F_1 = +4.00$ D, the segment refractive index n_s, and the main lens refractive index n_m:

$$F_{1,s} \;=\; \frac{n_s - 1}{r_1} \;=\; \frac{n_s - 1}{\dfrac{n_m - 1}{F_1}} \;=\; \frac{n_s - 1}{n_m - 1} \times F_1 \;=\; \frac{1.65 - 1}{1.52 - 1} \times (+4) \;=\; +5.00\ \text{D}.$$

Hence, the power of the contact surface is

$$F_{con} \;=\; A + F_1 - F_{1,s} \;=\; 2.50 + 4.00 - 5.00 \;=\; +1.50\ \text{D}.$$

The radius r_c of the depression curve is the same as the radius r_{con} of the contact surface,

which is $\quad r_{con} \;=\; \dfrac{n_m - n_s}{F_{con}} \;=\; \dfrac{1.52 - 1.65}{+1.50} \;=\; -0.08667\ \text{m}.$

Hence, from figure 8.1(b), with air to the left of the depression curve and the main lens to its right, the power of the depression curve is

$$F_c \;=\; \frac{n_m - 1}{r_c} \;=\; \frac{1.52 - 1}{-0.08867} \;=\; -6.00\ \text{D}.$$

Rather than use first principles, one may use the easily derived formula $F_c = F_1 - Ak$, where k is the bifocal blank ratio given by

$$k \;=\; \frac{n_m - 1}{n_s - n_m} \;=\; \frac{1.52 - 1}{1.65 - 1.52} \;=\; 4$$

where n_m and n_s are the refractive indices of the main lens and the segment, respectively.

Thus, $\quad F_c = F_1 - Ak \;=\; (+4.00) - (2.50 \times 4) \;=\; -6.00\ \text{D}.$

Part (b)

When the lens is made on a +2.00 D base curve the thin lens toric transposition is

$$\frac{+2.00\ \text{DC} \times 180\ /\ +4.00\ \text{DC} \times 90}{-10.00\ \text{DS}} \;.$$

Except for A, the following symbols will be found in figure 8.2:

A = Addition
$\quad F_1$ = power of front surface in the distance portion
$\quad F_2$ = power of back surface in the distance and near portions
$\quad F_{2,s}$ = power of the back surface over the segment
$\quad F_{con}$ = power of the contact surface between the segment button and the main lens
$\quad n_m$ = main lens refractive index and n_s = segment refractive index.

As before, $\quad$ *Addition = Reading portion power – Distance portion power.*

So, $\quad A = (F_1 + F_{con} + F_{2,s}) - (F_1 + F_2) \;=\; F_{con} + F_{2,s} - F_2$.

Hence, $\quad F_{con} = A + F_2 - F_{2,s}$ $\qquad$ (3).

We know the Add $A = +2.50$ and the back surface power in the distance portion is $F_2 = -10.00$ D in figure 8.2, so we must now find $F_{2,s}$, the power of the back surface on the segment. The radius of this surface can be found from the distance portion power, thus

$$r_2 = \frac{n_2' - n_2}{F_2} = \frac{1 - 1.52}{-10.00} = +0.0520 \text{ m.}$$

Using this radius, we can calculate the back surface power of the segment. Since the refractive index is $n_s = 1.65$ to the left of this surface and air is to the right, the power is

$$F_{2,s} = \frac{1 - n_s}{r_2} = \frac{1 - 1.65}{+0.0520} = -12.50 \text{ D.}$$

Then, using equation (3),

$$F_{con} = A + F_2 - F_{2,s} = (+2.50) + (-10.00) - (-12.50) = +5.00 \text{ D}$$

Now, the radius of the contact surface is

$$r_c = \frac{n_s - n_m}{F_{con}} = \frac{1.65 - 1.52}{+5.00} = +0.260 \text{ m}$$

so, since $r_c = r_{con}$ (they are identical!), the power of the depression curve (in air) is

$$F_c = \frac{1 - n_m}{r_c} = \frac{1 - 1.52}{+0.0260} = -20.00 \text{ D.}$$

In a similar manner to the calculation in part (a), the power of the depression curve can be obtained by the short-cut route of using a derived equation as follows:

$$F_c = F_2 - Ak = (-10.00) - (2.50 \times 4.00) = -20.00 \text{ D}$$

the bifocal blank ratio k being the same as in part (a).

---

2   **The prescription of a fused bifocal lens is $+2.00 / +1.00 \times 60$, addition $+3.00$ D. It is made on a -7.00 D base curve using glasses of refractive index $n_m = 1.52$ for the main lens and $n_s = 1.65$ for the segment. If the segment is 24 mm round, calculate the maximum thickness of the flint glass portion (the segment).**

The lens, transposed to its negative cyl form, is $+3.00 / -1.00 \times 150$. Obtaining the thin lens toric transposition is always a little easier if the sph/cyl transposition has the same sign for the cylinder as that given for the base curve. Here the base curve is -7.00 D so the sph/cyl transposition should have a minus cyl. Hence, the distance portion surfaces are

$$\frac{+10.00 \text{ DS}}{-7.00 \text{ DC} \times 60 / -8.00 \text{ DC} \times 150}.$$

We must find AB in figure 8.3(a). Two methods will be employed: one from first principles and the other by derived equations.

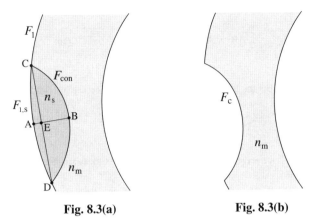

| Fig. 8.3(a) | Fig. 8.3(b) |

Method 1 — from first principles

AE and EB are the sags of the surfaces comprising the segment in figure 8.3(a). We must find these and add them together to arrive at AB, the segment thickness. We therefore need the radii of these surfaces. Using the power of the front surface in the distance portion,

$$r_1 = \frac{n_1' - n_1}{F_1} = \frac{1.52 - 1}{+10.00} = +0.052 \text{ m} = +52.0 \text{ mm}.$$

The power of the depression curve is $F_c = F_1 - Ak$, where k is the bifocal blank ratio given by

$$k = \frac{n_m - 1}{n_s - n_m} = \frac{1.52 - 1}{1.65 - 1.52} = 4$$

where n_m and n_s are the refractive indices of the main lens and the segment, respectively.

Thus, $F_c = F_1 - Ak = (+10) - (3 \times 4) = -2.00 \text{ D}.$
We can now find the radius (r_c) of the depression curve:

$$r_c = \frac{n_m - 1}{F_c} = \frac{1.52 - 1}{-2.00} = -0.260 \text{ m} = -260 \text{ mm}.$$

Next, we can calculate the sags of the two segment surfaces:

$$AE = r_1 - \sqrt{r_1^2 - y^2} = 52 - \sqrt{52^2 - 12^2} = 52 - 50.6 = 1.4 \text{ mm}$$

where y is half the diameter of the segment.

Then, $EB = r_c - \sqrt{r_c^2 - y^2} = 260 - \sqrt{260^2 - 12^2} = 260 - 259.7 = 0.3 \text{ mm}.$

(Recall that we obtained −260 mm for the radius r_c and note that the minus sign of the radius of curvature is not applied in this last step; this equation does not allow use of the sign convention.)

Then, the maximum thickness of the segment is

$$AB = AE + EB = 1.4 + 0.3 = 1.7 \text{ mm.}$$

It is worth mentioning that had we used the approximate sag formula $s = \dfrac{y^2 |F|}{2000 (n - 1)}$
to calculate the sags, the answer would have been 1.66 mm, which rounds to the same answer.

Method 2 — a derived equation using the approximate sag formula

Since the accurate and approximate sag formulas give the same answer to one decimal place, it is possible to use the following method. Figure 8.3(c) illustrates the idea.

F_s is the thin lens power of the segment in air and it can be shown that $F_s = A(k + 1)$ where A is the addition and k is the bifocal blank ratio. Therefore, in this question we have

$$F_s = A(k + 1) = 3 \times (4 + 1) = +15 \text{ D.}$$

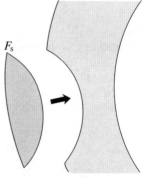

Fig. 8.3(c)

Since we have assumed thin lens theory for the power of the segment in air, we can ignore the form of the segment and assume it to be plano-convex, in which case its centre thickness is the sag of the convex surface of power F_s . This is given by the approximate sag formula. Writing t_s instead of s for the centre thickness of the segment, then

$$t_s = \frac{y^2 |F_s|}{2000 (n_s - 1)} = \frac{12^2 \times 15}{2000 \times (1.65 - 1)} = 1.66 \text{ mm.}$$

3 A fused bifocal is surfaced to produce the following prescription on a -6.00 D base curve: $+3.00 / +2.00 \times 90$. The depression curve is -5.00 DS. (i) Find the refractive index of the flint glass if the main lens is made of glass of refractive index 1.523, and (ii) calculate the addition if the blank ratio is 4.

(i) The blank ratio is defined as $k = \dfrac{n_m - 1}{n_s - n_m}$. We can rearrange this equation to give

the refractive index n_s of the segment glass. Thus,

$$(n_s - n_m)k = n_m - 1$$
$$\Rightarrow \quad n_s k - n_m k = n_m - 1$$
$$\Rightarrow \quad n_s k = n_m k + n_m - 1$$

$$\Rightarrow \qquad n_s = \frac{n_m k + n_m - 1}{k} = \frac{(1.523 \times 4) + 1.523 - 1}{4} = 1.654.$$

(ii) The addition can be calculated using the expression for the depression curve power F_c ; that is, $F_c = F_1 - Ak$, where A is the addition and k is the bifocal blank ratio.

Rearranging this expression to give the addition, $A = \dfrac{F_1}{k} - \dfrac{F_c}{k}$. Interestingly, note that

the first term on the right hand side gives the addition due to the front surface of the segment and the second term, including the minus sign, gives the addition due to the contact surface.

We must first find the front surface power (F_1) in the distance portion by writing the thin lens toric transposition:

$$\frac{+11.00 \text{ DS}}{-6.00 \text{ DC} \times 90 \, / \, -8.00 \text{ DC} \times 180}.$$

Hence, $F_1 = +11.00$ DS , and the addition is $A = \dfrac{F_1}{k} - \dfrac{F_c}{k} = \dfrac{11}{4} - \dfrac{(-5)}{4} = +4.00$ D.

---

4 A fused D segment trifocal is made to the following specification Rx $-3.00 / -2.00 \times 180$, Add $+2.50$ for near. It is made from the following glasses
    Main lens $n_m = 1.5300$ Intermediate segment $n_i = 1.5830$
    Reading segment $n_r = 1.6625$
in toric form with a -7.00 D base curve. What is the power of the depression curve, and what is the intermediate addition?

From figure 8.4, it can be seen that the curvature of the depression curve is the same in both portions of the segment. Hence, its power can be found by the same method as with a fused bifocal. It should also be mentioned that there are two blank ratios on this type of trifocal:

$$\text{Intermediate blank ratio } k_i = \frac{n_m - 1}{n_i - n_m} = \frac{1.5300 - 1}{1.5830 - 1.5300} = 10$$

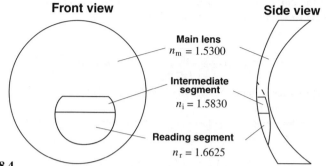

Front view

Side view

Main lens
$n_{\mathrm{m}} = 1.5300$

Intermediate
segment
$n_{\mathrm{i}} = 1.5830$

Reading segment
$n_{\mathrm{r}} = 1.6625$

Fig. 8.4

and the reading blank ratio $k_r = \dfrac{n_{\mathrm{m}} - 1}{n_r - n_{\mathrm{m}}} = \dfrac{1.5300 - 1}{1.6625 - 1.5300} = 4$.

The thin lens toric transposition of the distance portion is $\dfrac{+4.00}{-7.00 \times 90 \,/\, -9.00 \times 180}$.

That is, the front surface power of the distance portion is $F_1 = +4.00$ D.

We can find the power (F_{c}) of the depression curve using $F_{\mathrm{c}} = F_1 - Ak$, taking care that the correct value of k is used with the corresponding known addition, here the reading Add A_r.

So, $\qquad F_{\mathrm{c}} = F_1 - Ak = (+4) - (2.5 \times 4) = -6.00$ D.

Knowing F_{c} and k_{i}, we can find the intermediate addition as follows:

$$A_{\mathrm{i}} = \frac{F_1 - F_{\mathrm{c}}}{k_{\mathrm{i}}} = \frac{(+4) - (-6)}{10} = +1.00 \text{ D}.$$

---

5   The prescription R. +2.00 / +3.00 x 90, Add +2.00, is made up as a round segment
     bifocal with the optical centre of the segment coinciding with its geometrical centre.
     The segment specification is 24 x 3 below x 2 inset. The optical centre of the distance
     portion is 2 mm above the datum centre. Find the prismatic effect at a near visual
     point (NVP) which is 8 mm below and 2 mm in from the datum centre.

We shall continue to use the Datum System, along with the Boxed System, since it is still almost exclusively used in UK practice.

Problems of this nature are best solved by treating the lens as if it consisted of two separate components, the main lens and the segment. The prismatic effects produced by these portions are calculated separately and added together at the end. Firstly, however, it is necessary to determine the position of the visual point relative to each optical centre in turn; that is, relative to the optical centre (O_D) of the distance portion and the optical centre (O_S) of the segment. This can be done by sketching the main features of the lens and then locating the near visual point. From figure 8.5(a), it can be seen that relative to O_D the NVP is 10 mm below and 2 mm in, and relative to O_S the NVP is 7 mm vertically above it.

Prismatic effect due to distance portion

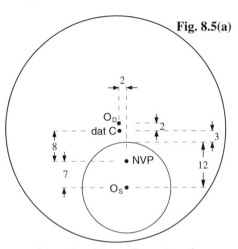

Fig. 8.5(a)

Since the cylinder axis is vertical, the distance portion power is that due to the sphere alone (+2.00 D) in the vertical meridian, so

$$P_V = c_V|F_V| = 1.0 \times 2 = 2^\Delta \text{ base up.}$$

The base direction can be obtained in several ways. One way is by drawing a vertical section through O_D which shows that the distance portion produces base up effect at the NVP; see the upper part of figure 8.5(b).

Dimensions in mm. Drawn to scale.

The distance portion power in the horizontal meridian is +5.00, so

$$P_H = c_H|F_H| = 0.2 \times 5 = 1.0^\Delta \text{ base out.}$$

This time the base direction is found by inspection of the lower part of figure 8.5(b).

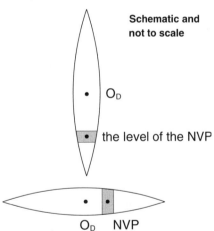

Fig. 8.5(b) Sections through O_D in the distance portion.

Prismatic effect due to the segment

$$P_V = c_V|F_V| = 0.7 \times 2 = 1.4^\Delta \text{ base down.}$$

The base direction can be obtained by inspection of figure 8.5(c) which shows a vertical section through the segment. There is no horizontal prismatic effect due to the segment because the NVP lies vertically above O_S .

The total prismatic effect at the NVP is obtained by adding the individual effects:

Fig. 8.5(c) Section through the segment.

103

$$P_V = 2^\Delta \text{ base up} + 1.4^\Delta \text{ base down} = 0.6^\Delta \text{ base up.}$$

$$P_H = 1.0^\Delta \text{ base out.}$$

---

6 **The prescription R. +5.00 / +2.00 x 90, addition +2.00, is to be made as a visible centre controlled bifocal with a 22 mm diameter segment. The segment drop (or cut) is 3 mm, and the segment centre is 2 mm inset. What single prism must be worked on the segment if there is to be no prismatic effect at the near visual point 10 mm down and 2 mm in from the distance optical centre?**

In figure 8.6(a), before prism is worked on the segment, at the near visual point N there are horizontal and vertical prismatic effects due to the distance portion, and a vertical prismatic effect due to the segment being vertically below N.

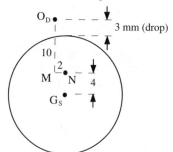

So, before prism is worked, the prismatic effect at N is:

Prismatic effect due to the distance portion

horizontal prism = MN × horizontal power
        $= 0.2 \times 7 = 1.4^\Delta$ base out.

vertical prism = MO_D × vertical power
        $= 1.0 \times 5 = 5^\Delta$ base up.

G_S = geometric centre of segment
O_D = distance optical centre
N = NVP

Prismatic effect due to the segment

Fig. 8.6(a)

vertical prism = NG_S × vertical power $= 0.4 \times 2 = 0.8^\Delta$ base down.

Therefore, the total prismatic effect at N is

vertically, 5^Δ base up + 0.8^Δ base down = 4.2^Δ base up.
horizontally, 1.4^Δ base out.

Combining these into a single prismatic effect, P, in figure 8.6(b) we have

Fig. 8.6(b)

$$P = \sqrt{4.2^2 + 1.4^2} = 4.43^\Delta$$

and $\theta = \arctan \dfrac{4.2}{1.4} = 71.6°$

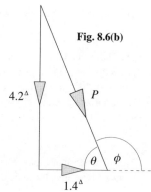

which makes $\phi = 180° - 71.6° = 108.4°.$
Hence, the resultant prismatic effect at N, before prism is worked, is 4.43^Δ base up 108.4°. To negate this, prism 4.43^Δ base down 108.4° must be worked.

104

7   The prescription R. −5.00 / +2.00 x 90, Add +2.00, is to be glazed as a D segment bi-
    prism (slab-off) bifocal with a segment 22 mm × 16 mm. the distance optical centre is
    at the centre of the circular uncut, and 5 mm above the segment top. The optical centre
    of the segment is 5 mm below the segment top, and the vertical prismatic effect is to be
    zero at that point. The uncut size is 60 mm round and the refractive index of the main
    lens is 1.5. Find the difference in thickness between the upper and lower extremities of
    the uncut.

Figure 8.7(a) shows the D segment bifocal without a slabbed-off portion. Since the lens is
regarded as being thin, we can make the lens in a more convenient form for the solution of
this problem. The most convenient form is with $F_1 = 0$ as shown in figure 8.7(b).

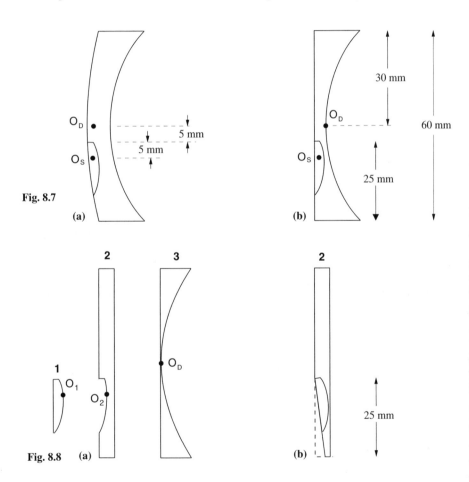

Figure 8.8(a) shows the new form of the lens 'exploded' into its components. O_1 and O_2 are the
optical centre of the segment and the depression components. The prismatic effect on the
whole lens at a point at the level of O_S (O_1 and O_2 are at the same level), see figure 8.7(a), is
due entirely to the exploded component 3. the optical centre of this component is 10 mm above

O_S and the power of this component in the vertical meridian, from the distance Rx, is −5 D. Using Prentice's Rule, this contributes $c|F| = 1.0 \times 5 = 5^\Delta$ base down at the level of O_S. The base direction at the level of O_1 and O_2 can be seen from component 3 in figure 8.8(a). This prism base down can be removed from component 2 by slabbing-off this amount. In effect, the front surface of the lens is tilted.

The distance from the top of the segment to the bottom edge of the uncut is 25 mm; see figure 8.7(b). We use the prism edge thickness difference formula to find the thickness of the base of the slabbed-off prism:

$$g = \frac{Pd}{100(n-1)} = \frac{5 \times 25}{100 \times (1.5-1)} = 2.5 \text{ mm}.$$

Therefore, the lower extremity of the uncut is 2.5 mm less thick than the upper extremity.

---

8   **The prescription −3.00 DS, Add +2.50, is made up as a standard 38 mm round segment bifocal. What is the jump?**

Jump may be defined as the sudden introduction of base down prism at the segment top. If the distance from the segment top to the optical centre of the segment is known, together with the addition, the magnitude of the jump can be calculated using Prentice's Rule. In this case (and in nearly all round segment bifocals),

Jump $(^\Delta)$ = *segment radius* (cm) × *Add* = $1.9 \times 2.5 = 4.75^\Delta$ (base down).

On looking downwards, as the vertical axis crosses the upper edge of the segment the patient sees a sudden angular displacement of the image through this amount (the jump).

---

9   **The prescription +4.00 /−2.00 x 180, Add +2.00, is made up as a bifocal with a standard 24 mm round segment. The segment top is 2 mm below the optical centre of the distance portion. Find the position of the optical centre (O_N) of the reading portion.**

This is most easily achieved using the equation $x = \dfrac{sA}{A+F}$ given by Jalie[†] in paragraph

86, where, in figure 8.9
O_D	is the optical centre of the distance portion
x	is the vertical distance from O_N to O_D
O_S	is the optical centre of the segment
s	is the vertical distance from O_D to O_S
F	is the power of the distance portion (in the vertical meridian)
A	is the addition.

In this case, the vertical power in the distance portion is +2.00 D, the addition is +2.00, $s = 14$ mm (segment radius 12 mm plus the drop 2 mm).

† Principles of Ophthalmic Lenses, Jalie, M., ABDO.

Hence

$$x = \frac{sA}{A+F} = \frac{14 \times 2}{2+2} = 7 \text{ mm.}$$

That is, the optical centre of the reading portion is 7 mm below the optical centre of the distance portion.

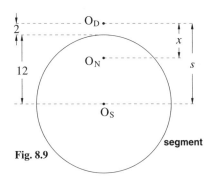

Fig. 8.9

---

10 The prescription R. +3.00 / +2.00 x 60, Add +2.00, is made up as an invisible solid bifocal with the distance optical centre 2 mm above the datum centre. The segment details are 22 × 3 below × 2 inset.

(a) Find the jump at the top of the segment.

(b) Find the position of the point in the reading portion at which there is no prismatic effect.

(a) From figure 8.10(a), we can see that at the top of the segment, T, the prismatic effect introduced by the segment is base down. The jump introduced at the top of the segment is the prismatic effect experienced due to the addition and the type of segment. The segment top is 1.1 cm above the geometrical (and optical) centre of the segment. Thus, using Prentice's Rule, the jump is $P = c |F| = 1.1 \times 2 = 2.2^{\Delta}$ base down.

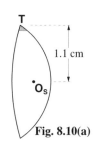

Fig. 8.10(a)

Since the distance optical centre, O_D, is 2 mm above datum and the segment top is 3 mm below datum, the segment top is 5 mm below the distance optical centre (i.e. the drop is 5 mm). The segment optical centre, O_S, is half the segment diameter, 11 mm, below the segment top. Therefore, O_S is $11 + 5 = 16$ mm below O_D, and 2 mm inset. Thus, in figure 8.10(b),

Fig. 8.10(b)

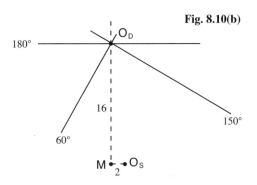

$O_D M = 16$ mm and $MO_S = 2$ mm.

Since the positions of O_D and O_S are responsible for prismatic effects within the reading portion, their effects must cancel at the near optical centre, O_N. Let O_N have a coordinate $O_DR = x$ along the 150° meridian with respect to O_D, and a coordinate $RO_N = y$ along the 60° meridian; see figure 8.10(c).

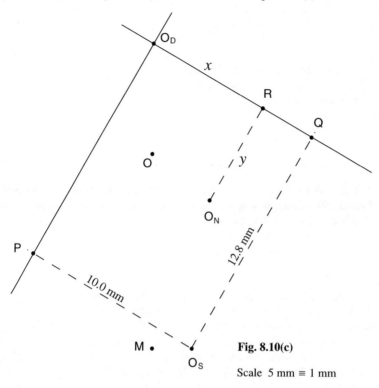

Fig. 8.10(c)

Scale 5 mm ≡ 1 mm

Along the 60° meridian

The prismatic effect at O_N due to the distance Rx is $c|F| = y \times 3 = 3y$ (y in cm)   (1).

The prismatic effect at O_N due to the segment is

$$c|F| = (QO_S - y) \times Add = (1.28 - y) \times 2 = 2.56 - 2y \qquad (y \text{ in cm}) \qquad (2).$$

These prismatic effects must be equal in magnitude but opposite in base direction for O_N to be the near optical centre (that is, free of any prismatic effect).   So, Equating (1) and (2),

$3y = 2.56 - 2y$, which leads to $5y = 2.56$, so $y = 0.512 \text{ cm} = 5.12 \text{ mm}$.

Along the 150° meridian

The prismatic effect at O_N due to the distance Rx is $c|F| = x \times 5 = 5x$ (x in cm)   (3).

The prismatic effect at O_N due to the segment is

$$c\,|F| = (PO_S - x) \times Add = (1.0 - x) \times 2 = 2 - 2x \qquad (4).$$

Equating (3) and (4), $5x = 2 - 2x$, which leads to $7x = 2$, so that $x = 0.29$ cm $= 2.9$ mm.

So, the near optical centre is 2.9 mm down the 150° meridian and 5.12 mm down the 60° meridian from O_D. In figure 8.10(c), which is drawn to scale, the point O represents the true position of O_N and measurement shows OO_S to be less than 11 mm, so that O_N (or O) is within the segment.

---

11 **Show that a vertical differential prismatic effect, ΔP, at the near visual points (NVP) on the lenses of an anisometropic prescription for bifocals can be eliminated if the difference in round segment diameters is $\Delta d = 20\, \Delta P\, /\, Add$ mm.**

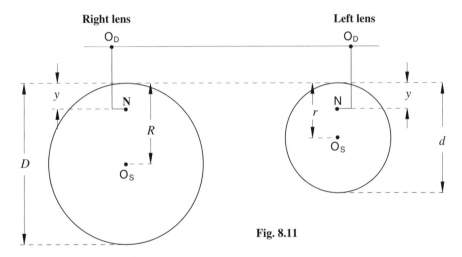

Fig. 8.11

Let the NVPs (shown as the points N) be a distance y below the segment tops and the segment radii be R and r (all measurements in cm). Then, using Prentice's Rule, $P = c\,|F|$, the prismatic effect at the NVPs due to the segments are

R. $\quad NO_S \times Add = (R - y) \times Add \qquad$ and $\qquad$ L. $\quad NO_S \times Add = (r - y) \times Add$.

These prismatic effects are vertical. Hence, the vertical differential prismatic effect at the NVPs due to the segments is $\quad \Delta P = (R - y) \times Add - (r - y) \times Add = (R - r) \times Add$.
But, $R - r = \frac{1}{2}(D - d)$, from figure 8.11, where D and d are the segment diameters, so writing $\Delta d = D - d$, the difference in the segment diameters, we have $\quad \Delta P = \frac{1}{2} \Delta d \cdot Add$

which gives $\qquad \Delta d = 2\dfrac{\Delta P}{Add}$ cm, $\qquad$ or $\qquad \Delta d = 20\dfrac{\Delta P}{Add}$ mm.

Thus, to find the required segment diameters in this type of problem, or in practice, is a simple matter once the vertical differential prismatic effect has been determined.

12 Given the table below, find the vertical differential prismatic effect ΔP at the near visual points 10 mm below and 2 mm in from the distance optical centres of the prescription   R. −2.00 / −1.75 x 65   L. −3.50 / −1.25 x 110   Add +2.00 and determine the difference in the round segment diameters to neutralize it.

Vertical prismatic effect at the NVP, 10 mm down and 2 mm in from the distance optical centre due to a +1.00 D cylinder. All base directions are UP. Reverse the base direction for minus cylinders.
Values for other cylinder powers can be obtained by multiplying by that cylinder power.

Axis	RE	LE	Axis	RE	LE
5	1.00	0.97	95	0.00	0.02
10	1.00	0.93	100	0.00	0.06
15	0.98	0.88	105	0.01	0.11
20	0.94	0.81	110	0.05	0.18
25	0.89	0.74	115	0.10	0.25
30	0.83	0.66	120	0.16	0.33
35	0.76	0.57	125	0.23	0.42
40	0.68	0.48	130	0.31	0.51
45	0.60	0.40	135	0.39	0.60
50	0.51	0.31	140	0.48	0.68
55	0.42	0.23	145	0.57	0.76
60	0.33	0.16	150	0.66	0.83
65	0.25	0.10	155	0.74	0.89
70	0.18	0.05	160	0.81	0.94
75	0.11	0.01	165	0.88	0.98
80	0.06	0.00	170	0.93	1.00
85	0.02	0.00	175	0.97	1.00
90	0.00	0.00	180	1.00	1.00

Vertical prismatic effect due to spheres

R. $P = c\,|F| = 1.0 \times |-2| = 2^\Delta$ base down
L. $P = c\,|F| = 1.0 \times |-3.5| = 3.5^\Delta$ base down.

Vertical prismatic effect due to cylinders

R. Due to a −1.00 D cyl axis 65° $= 0.25^\Delta$ base down
Due to a −1.75 D cyl axis 65° $= 1.75 \times 0.25^\Delta = 0.44^\Delta$ base down.

L. Due to a −1.00 D cyl axis 110° $= 0.18^\Delta$ base down
Due to a −1.25 D cyl axis 110° $= 1.25 \times 0.18^\Delta = 0.23^\Delta$ base down.

Total prismatic effect in each lens

R. 2^Δ base down + 0.44^Δ base down = 2.44^Δ base down
L. 3.5^Δ base down + 0.23^Δ base down = 3.73^Δ base down.

The vertical differential prismatic effect is ΔP = 3.73^Δ – 2.44^Δ = 1.29^Δ base down L.

The difference in segment diameters is Δd = $20 \times \dfrac{\Delta P}{Add}$ = $20 \times \dfrac{1.29}{2.00}$ = 12.9 mm.

Round segments, R. 45 mm and L. 30 mm, would most nearly satisfy this, with the larger segment in the right lens to add extra base down so that the extra base down from the distance portion in the left lens is neutralized.

---

13 **The following prescription is to be dispensed as bifocals:**
     R. –1.00 DS   L. –2.00 / –1.00 x 180   Add +2.00.
   (a) **What is the differential prismatic effect at near visual points 8 mm below the optical centres of the distance portion?**
   (b) **If a standard R24 mm segment were used for the left lens, what size segment for the right lens would eliminate the differential prismatic effect at the NVPs?**

(a) Differential prismatic effects have been dealt with in question 6.12. The approach here is exactly the same since the addition can be ignored (because differential prism is created by the distance prescription).

Thus, **Right Lens** P_V = $c_V \, |F_V|$ = $0.8 \times |-1|$ = 0.8^Δ base down.
The base direction is down since the optical centre is above the near visual point and the lens is minus.
     Left Lens P_V = $c_V \, |F_V|$ = $0.8 \times |-3|$ = 2.4^Δ base down.

The difference between these two prismatic effects is 1.6^Δ base down left.

(b) The difference in round segment diameters which would be required to overcome this amount of differential prism can be obtained using the expression

$$d_1 - d_2 = \frac{2c(F_1 - F_2)}{A}$$ which is equivalent to equation $\Delta d = 20 \times \dfrac{\Delta P}{Add}$ in question 12,

where
$d_1 - d_2$ is the difference in round segment diameters,
$F_1 - F_2$ is the difference between the R and L distance portion powers in the vertical meridian,
c is the vertical distance from the distance optical centre O_D to the near visual point,
and A is the addition.

Hence, $$d_1 - d_2 = \frac{2c(F_1 - F_2)}{A} = \frac{2 \times 8[(-1)-(-3)]}{2} = 16 \text{ mm.}$$

Therefore, if the segment before the left eye is a 24 mm round one, the segment required by the right eye would be 24 + 16 = 40 mm.

14 Solid invisible bifocal lenses are used for the prescription
   R. +1.25 / +3.00 x 180   L. −0.25 / −2.00 x 90   Add +2.00.
The lenses are centred for distance on datum. One segment is R22 mm and the other R45 mm. The segment tops are set 2 mm below datum. Calculate the position below datum common to both lenses where there is no vertical differential prism.

The point required on each lens is where the vertical differential prism due to the distance portions is cancelled by the vertical differential prism due to the segments. Let this point be N, in figure 8.12. In symbols then $\Delta P_{V,\,dist} = \Delta P_{V,\,segs}$.

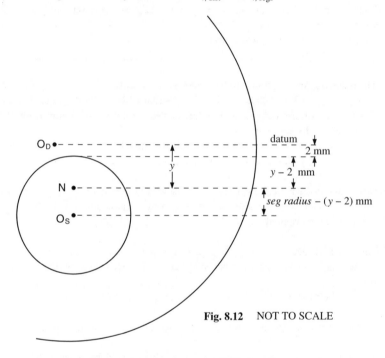

Fig. 8.12   NOT TO SCALE

Now, differentiating Prentice's Rule, $\Delta P = c \bullet \Delta F$, where ΔF is the vertical differential power, and writing $c = y$ from the diagram, we have

$$\Delta P_{V,\,dist} = y \bullet \Delta F = y \bullet 4.5 \quad or \quad \Delta P_{V,\,dist} = 4.5y \,.$$

Note that y is in cm and that $\Delta F = (F_R - F_L) = (+4.25) - (-0.25) = 4.5$ D.

For y in cm, we have $\qquad \Delta P_{V,\,dist} = y \bullet \Delta F = y \times 4.5 = 4.5y \qquad (1).$

The vertical differential prismatic effect due to the segments can be obtained from the equation $\Delta d = 20 \times \dfrac{\Delta P}{Add}$ which, with the addition of the subscripts, rearranges to give

$$\Delta P_{V,\,segs} = \frac{\Delta d \times Add}{20} = \frac{(45 - 22) \times 2}{20} = 2.3^{\Delta} \qquad (2).$$

Then equating the right hand sides of equations (1) and (2), since the left hand sides are equal, we arrive at

$$4.5y = 2.3 \qquad \text{or} \qquad y = \frac{2.3}{4.5} = 0.51 \text{ cm} = 5.1 \text{ mm.}$$

Alternative Method

The expression used to calculate the difference in segment diameters to eliminate vertical differential prism in anisometropia (see question 13) can also be used to solve this problem.

That is, $d_1 - d_2 = \dfrac{2c(F_1 - F_2)}{A}$

where here
$d_1 - d_2$ is the difference in round segment diameters,
$F_1 - F_2$ is the difference between the R and L distance portion powers in the vertical meridian,
c is the vertical distance from the distance optical centre O_D to the near visual point,
and A is the addition.

Rearranging the equation to make c the subject,

$$c = \frac{A(d_1 - d_2)}{2(F_1 - F_2)} = \frac{2 \times (45 - 22)}{2 \times (4.25 - (-0.25))} = 5.1 \text{ mm.}$$

That is, the point lies 5.1 mm below the optical centre of the distance portion.

---

15 **A no-jump bifocal is made to the prescription −4.00 / −1.00 x 90, Add +2.50. What prismatic effect would be encountered at a near visual point 8 mm below and 4 mm in from the optical centre of the distance portion? The segment drop is 2 mm and the geometric inset is also 2 mm.**

From figure 8.13, it can be seen that relative to the optical centre of the distance portion, the NVP is 8 mm below and 4 mm in (given) and, that relative to the optical centre (O_S) of the segment, it can be deduced that the NVP is 6 mm below and 2 mm in. As in question 5, we can now calculate the prismatic effect due to the main lens and segment separately, and add them together.

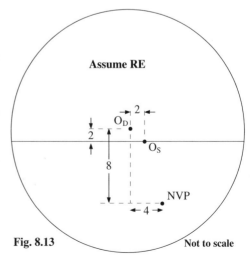

Fig. 8.13

113

Prismatic effect due to the distance portion:

Using F_V and F_H for the vertical and horizontal distance portion powers, respectively,

$P_V = c_V |F_V| = 0.8 \times 4 = 3.2^\Delta$ base down and $P_H = c_H |F_H| = 0.4 \times 5 = 2.0^\Delta$ base in.

Prismatic effect due to the segment:

Using F_A for the Add,

$P_V = c_V |F_A| = 0.6 \times 2.5 = 1.5^\Delta$ base up and $P_H = c_H |F_A| = 0.2 \times 2.5 = 0.5^\Delta$ base out.

The total prismatic effect is obtained by adding the individual amounts:

$$P_V = 3.2^\Delta \text{ base down} + 1.5^\Delta \text{ base up} = 1.7^\Delta \text{ base down}$$

$$P_H = 2.0^\Delta \text{ base in} + 0.5^\Delta \text{ base out} = 1.5^\Delta \text{ base in.}$$

9   PROTECTIVE LENSES

1   **What is the electromagnetic spectrum? Pay particular attention to those regions of importance to the optician.**

The electromagnetic spectrum is the entire distribution of electromagnetic waves according to their frequency or wavelength. In vacuum, all electromagnetic waves travel with the same speed of 2.99793×10^8 ms^{-1}. The whole spectrum covers a wide range of frequencies and subsections bear different names. These different names reflect the emission, transmission and absorption characteristics of the corresponding waves. However, there is no precise agreement on where one bandwidth starts and another finishes. There is therefore some overlap.

The entire spectrum from the lowest to the highest frequency (longest to the shortest wavelength) includes radio waves, microwaves, infrared (heat) radiation, visible light, ultraviolet radiation, X-rays, gamma rays and cosmic electromagnetic rays.

If c is the velocity of electromagnetic radiation in vacuum, ν (nu) is the frequency, and λ (lambda) is the wavelength, the fundamental relationship between these quantities is $c = \nu\lambda$. Clearly, since the speed of light is constant in vacuum, the higher frequencies are coupled with shorter wavelengths.

The energy associated with each photon (wave packet) of an electromagnetic radiation is given by $E = h\nu$, where ν is the frequency and h is is Planck's constant (6.63×10^{-34} Joule seconds (Js)). Thus, the higher the frequency the greater the energy per photon.

The bands of electromagnetic radiation of interest to opticians and optometrists are the ultraviolet, the visible and the infrared regions.

Ultraviolet (UV)

Adjacent to the visible spectrum but with shorter wavelengths (higher frequencies) is the ultraviolet band. The wavelengths range from about 1 nm to 390 nm and the corresponding frequencies are 3.0×10^{17} Hz and 7.7×10^{14} Hz. It is divided into three regions according to the biological effects: UVC is from 1 nm to 280 nm, UVB from 280 nm to 315 nm, and UVA from 315 nm to 390 nm. Ultraviolet radiation from the sun has more than enough energy to ionise atoms in the upper atmosphere, and in so doing creates the ionosphere. These photon energies are also of the order of magnitude to initiate many chemical reactions. Fortunately, the ozone (O_3) in the atmosphere absorbs what would otherwise be a lethal stream of UV photons.

Sources of UV are hot bodies or excited gases. The UV photons are emitted when inner and outer electrons in atomic 'orbits' or shells fall back to lower energy levels, whilst satisfying the required frequency range for UV occurring in the equation $E = h\nu$. Hence, artificial sources as well as the sun produce UV. High temperature surfaces such as the sun produce a continuous spectrum of UV, whereas gaseous discharge tubes produce discrete spectral line emissions.

Infrared (IR)

Adjacent to the visible spectrum, on the long wavelength side, is the infrared band. The wavelengths range from 760 nm to 1 mm. At the long wavelength end, microwave oscillators will generate IR as well as incandescent sources. Any material will radiate or absorb IR via thermal agitation of its molecules. Continuous spectra are emitted by dense gases, liquids and solids, and specific narrow bands by thermally excited isolated molecules. The emissions arise from vibrations and rotations of molecules.

Light

The visible band of the electromagnetic spectrum extends from about 390 nm wavelength to 760 nm. It is produced by the outer electrons in atoms and molecules falling back to lower energy levels from higher excited states. In an incandescent material the electrons are accelerated randomly and undergo frequent collisions. This thermally excited radiation produces a broad, continuous spectrum. The tungsten bulb is perhaps the best known example of an artificial incandescent source.

In a gaseous discharge tube the light emitted is characteristic of the energy levels of the particular gas. The spectrum emitted consists of discrete bands or lines, as seen in the spectroscope. In the fluorescent tube used for lighting, the tube is filled with mercury vapour at a very low pressure. The electrons ejected from the electrodes collide with the mercury atoms, excite them (raise electrons to higher energy levels), and cause them to emit some discrete visible radiations, but mostly they emit UV. The UV strikes the fluorescent substance (zinc sulphide) coating the inner surface of the tube, which causes the coating to emit radiation in the visible spectrum.

---

2   Discuss the biological effects of ultraviolet, infrared and intense visible radiation on the eyes.

We shall consider the effects of each type of radiation separately.

The Effects of Ultraviolet Radiation

This radiation can be emitted from the sun, mercury vapour lamps and high intensity incandescent lamps. Sunlight is the most common source, but ultraviolet lamps are used for medical and dental purposes, and industrial purposes such as sterilisation.

The direct effects of UV exposure are limited to the surface of the skin since the rays are absorbed at or near the surface. Except where cancer occurs, the skin recovers from the effects which include sunburn (reddening), pigmentation (suntan), and progressive adaptation to heavier doses.

Reddening occurs in one to several hours and, depending on the exposure, it may be accompanied by tenderness, blisters, swelling, or sloughing of the outer layers of the skin. The outer skin cells may be damaged or destroyed, resulting in liberation from the cells of fluids and histamine (a nitrogen compound) into the surrounding tissues. Nerve cells in the skin react to the increased pressure and heat by signalling pain. UVB and UVC are absorbed by the cornea, but UVA penetrates the cornea to be absorbed by the crystalline lens. Chronic exposure to UVA radiation over several decades leads to the generation and accumulation of fluorescent chromophores responsible for the yellow coloration of the crystalline lens. This process, when advanced, produces brown nuclear cataract.

The eye cannot adapt to UV exposure. The wavelength range of UV radiation which causes sunburn, UVB, can also cause inflammation of the cornea accompanied by epithelial loss and subsequent severe pain. This is what happens in snowblindness or after exposure to strong UV sources. In addition to the process noted above, UVA radiation, the effects of which are cumulative in the crystalline lens, can also increase the rate at which senile cataract develops.

The energy of UV radiation is absorbed by raising the energy levels of 'orbital' electrons; an electron jumps to a higher energy level when an atom absorbs a photon, thereby placing the atom in a state of excitation whereupon it is more chemically active. UVB radiation is potentially more damaging than UVA because each photon contains more energy and can make the molecules in the skin more chemically reactive. Wavelengths below 295 nm do not reach the Earth's surface, although artificial sources do produce wavelengths below this level. Wavelengths of 220 nm are particularly toxic for cells.

The Effects of Infrared Radiation

The energy of IR radiation is absorbed by whole molecules and atoms. Overdosage of IR radiation, usually from direct exposure to a hot object or flame, can cause severe burns. IR wavelengths below 1400 nm (the infrared A or IRA region) can penetrate the cornea and have been responsible in the past for thermal cataract in glass blowers. Burns of the retina and choroid are possible from large doses of IR, usually coupled with visible light. Sunblindness (eclipse blindness) is caused by intense visible light and IR radiation producing irreversible bleaching of the visual pigments.

The Effects of Intense Visible Light

In ordinary intensities, visible light has no detrimental effects. Discomfort may be experienced, however, in excessive diffuse light or in the presence of intense localised direct or reflected light. Diffuse light, in excessive intensities, and coupled with surfaces possessing high reflectances produces veiling glare. There is an excessive bleaching of the visual pigment in the cones responsible for photopic vision. Consequently, the eye's sensitivity is reduced and the subject is aware of visual discomfort. Pain is associated with reflex contraction of the iris sphincter, and possibly with reflex dilatation of the conjunctival blood vessels. Reading a newspaper under a bright blue sky, or sunlight reflected from the paper, is a good example of veiling glare. A localised, excessively intense visible light close to an object of regard rapidly bleaches the visual pigments close to the foveola. By induction, this may markedly reduce the eye's sensitivity and in extreme cases make the subject temporarily blind. For example, looking directly into a photographer's flash-bulb will produce an after-image which may persist for a minute or so, during which time it will not be possible to read. Such glare is called scotomatic glare. Car headlights can cause a similar effect.

Lasers can generate intense visible light. Even the low power lasers used in teaching laboratories, such as the helium-neon laser of perhaps 300 mW power, can cause retinal burns if viewed directly by the eye. Higher power lasers, such as the carbon dioxide and solid state lasers, can cause severe injury even at a great distance. Pulsed lasers are even more hazardous because of their high peak intensities and because there is no chance to respond to the sudden flash. There is little hazard, however, when light from a low power continuous beam laser is used to illuminate a diffusing surface.

---

3   At a given wavelength the spectral transmittance, τ, for a 2 mm thick sample of ophthalmic glass is 0.6. If the refractive index is 1.5, find the transmittance of each surface and of the material. (N.B. It is conventional in modern physics to use T and R for transmittance and reflectance at lens surfaces. Hence, we shall use T_1 and T_2 for the transmittances of the two surfaces, and T_m for the transmittance of the material.)

The transmittances of the first and second surfaces are given by:

$$T_1 \ (= T_2) = \frac{4nn'}{(n' + n)^2} = \frac{4 \times 1 \times 1.5}{(1.5 + 1)^2} = 0.96, \ \text{for normal incidence.}$$

If T_m represents the fraction of the intensity leaving the first surface which reaches the second surface, we can find T_m from the relationship: *spectral transmittance* $= \tau = T_1 T_m T_2$.

$$\text{So,} \ \ T_m = \frac{\tau}{T_1 T_2} = \frac{0.6}{0.96 \times 0.96} = 0.651.$$

---

4   Define the terms *reflectance, transmittance, spectral transmittance* and *total transmittance*. A sample of ophthalmic glass 2 mm thick has $n = 1.5$ and a transmittance for the material, $T_m = 0.8$, for a particular wavelength of light. What percentage of the incident intensity (I_i) will leave the far surface of a sample 5 mm thick? Assume the incident beam is monochromatic, of the wavelength for which T_m is given, and the angle of incidence is $0°$.

At a boundary between two optical media, reflectance R is defined as the ratio of the reflected intensity to the incident intensity; in symbols $R = I_r / I_i$.

Transmittance T is the ratio of the transmitted intensity to the incident intensity on the surface. If the medium is non-absorbing, this fraction of the incident intensity on a first lens surface will reach the second surface.

The spectral transmittance is the ratio of the transmitted intensity (I_t) leaving the far surface to the intensity (I_i) incident upon the first surface. It is measured for each wavelength. In symbols, the spectral transmittance τ is $\tau = I_t / I_i$. Spectral transmittance represents the fraction of the incident intensity which is transmitted by the sample at each wavelength.

Total transmittance takes into account the spectrum of the incident light. Its definition is the same as for spectral transmittance except that it is the sum of all the transmitted intensities divided by the sum of all the incident intensities at each wavelength.

At the first surface in figure 9.1, let the incident intensity for the specified wavelength be I_i. A fraction T_1 of this will cross the first surface so that the intensity emerging from the first surface will be $T_1 I_i$. This will be attenuated by a factor T_m on traversing 2 mm of the glass, so the intensity 2 mm into the glass will be $T_1 T_m I_i$. After a further 2 mm the intensity will have been reduced further by another factor of T_m and will be $T_1 T_m^2 I_i$. Note that for each 2 mm of material the power on T_m is raised by 1. For a further 1 mm the power will be raised by ½, so after 5 mm the intensity will be $T_1 T_m^{2.5} I_i$. After passing through the second surface the intensity will be attenuated by the surface transmittance T_2, so the intensity (I_t) transmitted through the whole sample will be $T_1 T_m^{2.5} T_2 I_i$.

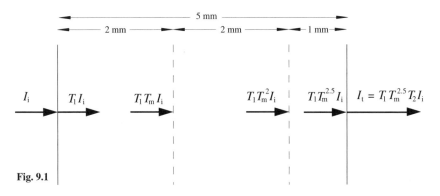

Fig. 9.1

Now, the surface transmittance T is given by $T = (4nn')/(n'-n)^2$ and for the first surface

this gives $T_1 = \dfrac{4nn'}{(n'+n)^2} = \dfrac{4 \times 1 \times 1.5}{(1.5+1)^2} = 0.96$, for normal incidence.

Then, by definition, the spectral transmittance is

$$\tau = \frac{I_t}{I_i} = \frac{T_1 T_m^{2.5} T_2 I_i}{I_i} = \frac{0.96 \times 0.8^{2.5} \times 0.96 \, I_i}{I_i} = 0.528 = 52.8\%$$

the I_i having cancelled. This is the fraction of the incident intensity which emerges from the second surface.

---

5   **Work question 4 using optical densities.**

The optical density of the 5 mm sample consists of the surface optical densities, which are equal, and the optical density of the 5 mm thickness of the medium. The latter is 2.5 times the optical density of a 2 mm thick sample. Now, the first surface optical density is

$$D_1 = \log \frac{1}{T_1} = \log \frac{1}{0.96} = 0.01773 .$$

Since $T_2 = T_1$, then $D_2 = D_1$, and the optical density of a 2 mm thick medium is

$$D_m = \log \frac{1}{T_m} = \log \frac{1}{0.8} = 0.09691 \; .$$

The total optical density D of the whole sample is

$$D = D_1 + (2.5 \times D_m) + D_2 \; = \; 0.01773 + (2.5 \times 0.09691) + 0.01773 \; = \; 0.27774 \; .$$

But $D = \log \dfrac{1}{\tau}$, so $\tau = \dfrac{1}{\text{antilog } D} = \dfrac{1}{1.8956} = 0.528$, again.

---

6 **Sketch the following transmittance curves:**
   (a) a neutral filter   **(b) a yellow contrast filter**
   (c) a UV absorbing filter   **(d) a heat absorbing filter.**
What colour would each tint have when viewing a white surface through it?

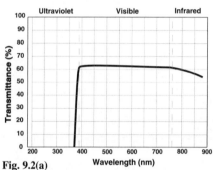

Fig. 9.2(a)

Figure 9.2(a) shows a neutral filter's transmittance curve. That part of the curve in the visible spectrum is approximately horizontal, indicating that the intensity at each wavelength is equally attenuated. As a result, all colours are reduced in luminosity by the same fractional amount so that a white surface would appear grey.

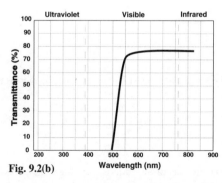

Fig. 9.2(b)

Figure 9.2(b) shows a contrast filter's transmittance curve. It has a cut-off at about 500 mm and appears yellow when viewing a white surface since it transmits green, yellow and red which 'mix' to give a subjective impression of yellow.

Figure 9.2(a) will suffice for a UV absorbing filter. The cut-off must not be below 380 nm, although many modern UV blockers on CR 39 lenses now have a cut-off at 400 nm. This takes into account modern day thinking on the effect of UVA on the crystalline lens and on the retina in aphakic eyes.

120

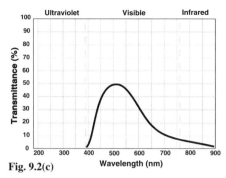
Fig. 9.2(c)

Figure 9.2(c) shows a heat-absorbing filter's transmittance curve. It appears blue-green since the visible red transmittance is low relative to the blue and green. Heat absorbing filters generally absorb in the UV range since heat sources output in the UV too.

Note that the colour of a filter gives a rough indication of which wavelengths are transmitted in the visible spectrum, but it says nothing about the UV and IR absorbing properties. Also, note that the contrast filter shown filters out blue and transmits the rest of the visible spectrum. Strictly, we could call it a blue filter or a yellow tint. In practice we use the word tint, together with the trade name, when describing a filter.

---

7   What is meant by luminous transmittance (*LT*). Include an explanation of its usefulness.

A transmittance curve for a tint is a plot of the Spectral Transmittances over the domain of the wavelengths measured, usually from 200 nm to 900 nm, although this may extend to 1400 nm. The sample for a solid tint (material tint) is usually 2 mm thick. From this graph we can see what happens at each wavelength. This is very important when we wish to see the absorption and transmission characteristics of a particular lens material. Spectral Transmittance curves are plotted on a spectrophotometer, the whole process being automated. Considering the visible spectrum alone, it is useful to have a single figure for comparing the relative darkening effects of tints. The Luminous Transmittance does this[†] and, indeed, allow us to compare the relative luminosities even for lenses with differently coloured tints. For example, if we look at a white surface through a green tint and then through a brown tint, both with a Luminous Transmittance of 60% say, then the surface will be equally reduced in brightness (luminosity) in both cases, even though appearing differently coloured.

The Luminous Transmittance is calculated as follows. Using a standard lamp with a known intensity emission $e(\lambda)$ for each wavelength in the visible spectrum, a standard eye's photopic spectral luminous efficiency function $V(\lambda)$, and the Spectral Transmittance values $\tau(\lambda)$ for the tint in question, two graphs are plotted. One is the graph of $e(\lambda)V(\lambda)$ and the other is $e(\lambda)\tau(\lambda)V(\lambda)$. For simplicity, these are written as eV and $e\tau V$.

Since $\tau < 1$, then $e\tau V < eV$. Hence, *area under* $e\tau V$ < *area under* eV.

The Luminous Transmittance is defined as $LT = \dfrac{area\ under\ e\tau V}{area\ under\ eV}$.

This gives the eye's judgement of the source's intensity with the filter (the numerator) compared with the eye's judgement of the source's intensity without the filter.

---

† In the case of contrast filters, there is a neuro-physiological effect which makes the scene viewed through the filter appear bright, even though the filter is aborbing some of the incident light. See *Introduction to Visual Optics*, page 439.

8 Write notes on (a) photochromic glass, (b) Transitions lenses, (c) Polaroid and similar materials, (d) toughened lenses.

(a) Photochromic glass darkens when irradiated by UV and visible light. The process is reversible so that removing the radiations causes the glass to become less dark, eventually returning to an almost untinted state. The action is due to the inclusion of silver chlorides, bromides or iodides, or a mixture of these in the glass material. Collectively, these compounds are known as silver halides. They form microscopic crystals dispersed throughout the glass.

The darkening effect is similar to the process taking place in photographic film. Light provides the energy to break the silver-halogen bond and form silver and halogen atoms. The silver atoms then absorb light, thus causing the glass to darken. However, unlike in photographic film, the halogen is not removed by chemical action and neither can it escape by diffusion. Hence, when the light is removed recombination of the silver and halogen takes place and the glass clears. Recombination is easier at higher temperatures, so the glass does not darken as much on warm days as it does on cold sunny days, although modern glasses are less sensitive in this respect. After 1 hour in the sun at 5°, 25° and 35°C, Photobrown Extra darkens to 19%, 24% and 36% transmittances, respectively.

Darkening (activation) is a quicker process than fading (clearing or bleaching). Photobrown Extra darkens to 30% transmittance within 60 seconds. On removal of the light, fading is a slower process, Photobrown Extra taking 20 minutes to clear to 70% transmittance, although it clears to 60% transmittance in under 5 minutes.

(b) Transitions is the name given to a plastic photochromic lens in which a surface imbibition process of photochromic material produces an equitint. The process is patented by Transitions Optical. It results in a 0.15 mm thick penetration of the lens material, compared with typically 0.01 mm depth for a conventional tint dye. It can be used on single vision, bifocal and multifocal lenses. The darkened state transmittance curve for Transitions Grey is

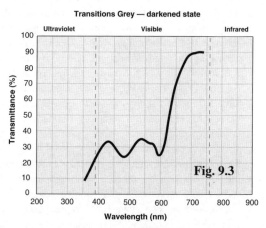

shown in figure 9.3. Transitions Eurobrown, Transitions III and Transitions XTRActive are more recent variations on the theme. With the exception of XTRActive, Transitions lenses darken to about 30% transmittance in less than 5 minutes and fade to 70% transmittance in about the same time at 22°C. The range for Transitions Eurobrown is 22% – 86% (at 22°C). XTRActive, a darker tint, ranges from about 12% to 63% at the same temperature. As with glass photochromics, they are somewhat temperature sensitive, darkening less at higher temperatures and more at lower ones. They do not darken inside a car.

(c) The modus operandi of Polaroid can be explained on a macroscopic scale by the wire-grid polariser, figure 9.4.

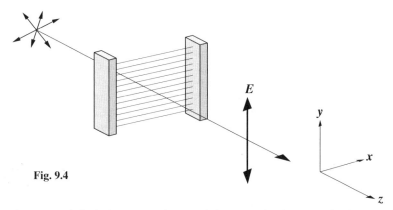

Fig. 9.4

Imagine an unpolarised electromagnetic wave (microwave, $\lambda = 1$ cm, say) impinges on the grid of horizontal copper wires stretched between two insulating blocks. The electric field can be resolved into two orthogonal components parallel to the wires (the x-axis) and perpendicular to the wires (the y-axis). The x-component drives the conduction electrons as an alternating current along the length of the wires, which transfers energy to the wires thereby heating them (joule heat). Also, electrons thus accelerated re-radiate in both the forward and backward directions, the latter appearing as a reflected wave. The forward re-radiation is dispersed, the result being little or no transmission of the x-component.

The y-component, however, loses little or no energy since the electrons are not free to move very far across the width of the wires. Thus, the y-component propagates through the grid hardly altered. We see then that the transmission axis is perpendicular to the wires.

Polaroid's mechanism is analagous to the wire-grid's. A sheet of clear polyvinyl alcohol is heated and stretched in a given direction. Its long hydrocarbon molecules become aligned and, when the sheet is dipped in a solution rich in iodine, the iodine attaches to the straight, long, chain-like molecules forming a molecular 'wire-grid'. The conduction electrons move along the 'chains' in the same manner as in the wire-grid. It is a very effective polariser across almost the entire visible spectrum, being somewhat less effective at the violet end where it is said to be 'leaky'. When viewing a very bright white light through crossed Polaroids there will be some leakage which appears dark violet.

(d) Untreated glass can fracture under stress into a multitude of sharp fragments. However, if a spectacle crown lens, for example, is heated to just below its softening temperature and suddenly chilled by jets of cold air, the sudden cooling of the surfaces renders them rigid before the interior. Contraction of the interior occurs on cooling, thus setting up a compressive stress in the surfaces. This compression must be overcome before the surface can fracture. If the surface is broken there is a release of a considerable amount of stored energy which propagates throughout the interior. This causes cracks in all directions and results in the 'heat tempered' or toughened lens breaking into characteristic small, cube-like fragments.

123

All cutting operations must be done before heat toughening (air tempering), otherwise they would initiate release of the stored energy. In order to withstand sufficient stress without shattering, the lens normally has to be made somewhat thicker than usual. Pilkington, however, has developed a heat tempering process with lenses of conventional thickness.

Chemically tempered glass is a more recent development. The compressive surface layer is provided by exchanging smaller ions in the glass for larger ones in a bath of molten salt. For example, if a glass rich in lithium ions is immersed in molten sodium chloride, many of the lithium ions escape and are replaced by the larger sodium ions. When the glass cools, the presence of the larger sodium ions creates a compressive stress in the surface. Lithium-rich glass may be used with either a sodium or a potassium salt bath; or, a sodium-rich glass may be used with a potassium salt bath. The size of the ions in ascending order is lithium, sodium and potassium.

---

9 **Discuss single layer and multilayer anti-reflection coatings on glass lenses. Calculate the reflectance at 555 nm when magnesium fluoride is used on glasses of refractive index 1.52 and 1.70. Explain why the bloom is a deeper purple on the 1.70 glass.**

One or more films of suitable materials deposited on a lens surface may be used to modify the reflectance and transmittance. Single films are used in single-layer anti-reflection coatings to reduce the reflectance, and in reflection filters to reduce the transmittance. Multilayer films are now the more common type in spectacle lenses since they have become reasonably inexpensive in the nineteen-nineties. They reduce the reflectance considerably more than do single layer ones.

Single layer anti-reflection (AR) coating

The conditions to be satisfied are called the *amplitude* and *path conditions*. In the amplitude condition, the amplitudes of the waves reflected from the air-film and the film-substrate boundaries should be equal. The path condition requires that the film should be one-quarter of a film-wavelength thick so that the two reflected waves are antiphase. For a single layer film these are satisfied when

$$n_f = \sqrt{n_s} \quad \text{and} \quad t = \frac{\lambda}{4n_f}$$

where n_f is the refractive index of the film material, n_s is the refractive index of the substrate (the glass), t is the thickness of the film and λ is the wavelength of the light. The wavelength chosen will be 555 nm for photopic vision and about 507 nm for scotopic vision. The former produces a magenta bloom (residual colour or reflex) and the latter produces a gold bloom.

Magnesium fluoride ($n_f = 1.38$) does not have the optimum refractive index for ophthalmic glasses but is used because of its durability. Assuming the variation in refractive index with wavelength does not affect the result significantly, the amplitude reflectances r_1 and r_2 at the air-film and film-substrate boundaries are, for normal incidence,

$$r_1 = -\left(\frac{n_f - 1}{n_f + 1}\right) = -\left(\frac{1.38 - 1}{1.38 + 1}\right) = -0.160$$

$$\text{and} \quad r_2 = -\left(\frac{n_s - n_f}{n_s + n_f}\right) = -\left(\frac{1.52 - 1.38}{1.52 + 1.38}\right) = -0.048.$$

The resultant amplitude reflectance is $r = |r_1| - |r_2| = 0.160 - 0.048 = 0.112$ and the intensity reflectance is $R = r^2 = 0.112^2 = 0.0125$. That is, 1.25% of the 555 nm light is reflected.

Repeating the calculation for $n_s = 1.70$, we have:

$$r_1 = -\left(\frac{n_f - 1}{n_f + 1}\right) = -\left(\frac{1.38 - 1}{1.38 + 1}\right) = -0.160, \text{ the same as before}$$

$$\text{and} \quad r_2 = -\left(\frac{n_s - n_f}{n_s + n_f}\right) = -\left(\frac{1.70 - 1.38}{1.70 + 1.38}\right) = -0.104.$$

This time, the resultant amplitude reflectance is $r = |r_1| - |r_2| = 0.160 - 0.112 = 0.056$ and the intensity reflectance is $R = r^2 = 0.056^2 = 0.0031$. That is, 0.31% of the 555 nm light is reflected. That is $0.31/1.25 = 0.248$ or about one-quarter of the amount of light reflected on the 1.52 index glass. Because less light at the centre of the visible spectrum is reflected from the coated 1.70 index glass, the residual colour is more saturated and appears a deeper magenta.

Multilayer coatings

One of the early multilayer coatings in the nineteen eighties was Hoya's three-layer film which resulted in more than 99% of the incident flux being transmitted by the lens. Figure 9.5 shows the schematic arrangement.

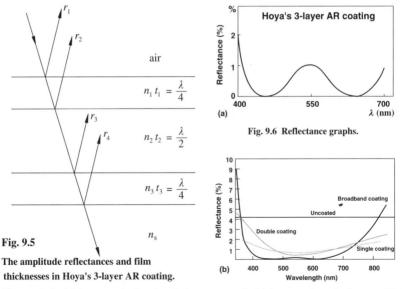

Fig. 9.5

The amplitude reflectances and film thicknesses in Hoya's 3-layer AR coating.

Fig. 9.6 Reflectance graphs.

The optical thicknesses (*refractive index* × *actual thickness*, *nt*) and the amplitude reflectances are indicated in the figure. r_1 and r_3, and r_2 and r_4 are in phase, but the two sets are made antiphase and they cancel for two wavelengths. The intensity reflectance versus wavelength is shown in figure 9.6(a). The bloom appears pale green because of the

125

preponderance of green in the reflection. As many as 6 or 7 layers are used nowadays to produce what is called a broadband AR coating. The layers are alternate low and high refractive index films and the coating is called broadband because the reflectance is less than 0.5% from each surface over a wide band of wavelengths from about 450 to 650 nm; see figure 9.6(b). It is now possible to achieve the same results on CR 39 and polyurethane (mid- and high index) plastics.

---

10   **The surfaces of a lens, $n_s = 1.50$ (s for substrate), are to be coated with magnesium fluoride, $n_f = 1.38$, so that a minimum reflection of $\lambda = 550$ nm will occur with normally incident light. Calculate (a) the reflectance for $\lambda = 550$ nm and (b) for 400 and 700 nm.**

(a) The calculations require the use of amplitude reflectances. Denoting these by r_1 and r_2 at the air-film and film-substrate boundaries, we have

$$r_1 = -\left(\frac{n_f - 1}{n_f + 1}\right) = -\left(\frac{1.38 - 1}{1.38 + 1}\right) = -0.1597$$

$$\text{and} \quad r_2 = -\left(\frac{n_s - n_f}{n_s + n_f}\right) = -\left(\frac{1.50 - 1.38}{1.50 + 1.38}\right) = -0.0417.$$

If the film thickness is $t = \dfrac{\lambda}{4n_f} = \dfrac{550}{4 \times 1.38} = 99.6$ nm, then the two reflected waves

will be antiphase and the resultant amplitude reflectance will be

$$r = |r_1| - |r_2| = 0.1597 - 0.0417 = 0.1180$$

and the intensity reflectance is $R = r^2 = 0.1180^2 = 0.0139 \approx 1.4\%$.

(Note that the minus sign for r_1 and r_2 indicates a π phase change on reflection).

(b) For other wavelengths the two reflected beams will not be antiphase. There will be some other phase change than π, since for these wavelengths the optical path differs from that for 550 nm. For $\lambda = 550$ nm, the optical path difference is twice the optical thickness; that is,

$$OPD = 2n_f t = 2 \times \frac{\lambda}{4} = 2 \times \frac{550}{4} = 275 \text{ nm}$$

which is half a vacuum wavelength, of course. However, for $\lambda = 400$ nm this optical thickness is 275/400 or 0.6875 of a wavelength. This represents a phase change of $0.6876 \times 2\pi$ radians, which is 247.5°. We can assume the refractive indices for the film and the substrate are near enough the same as for $\lambda = 550$ nm, but we cannot simply subtract the amplitude reflectances since the phase difference is not 180°. We must find the resultant r from a vector diagram in figure 9.7. r_1 and r_2 have the same magnitudes as before. We are assuming n_f has the same value for all wavelengths!

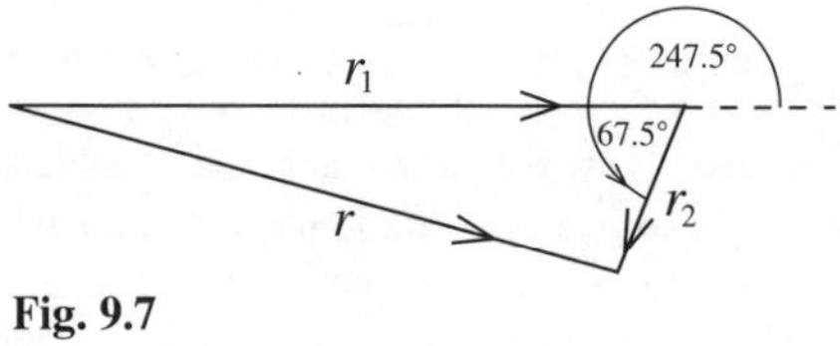

Fig. 9.7

Using the cosine rule, $r^2 = r_1{}^2 + r_2{}^2 - 2 r_1 r_2 \cos 67.5°$
$$= (0.1597)^2 + (0.0417)^2 - 2 \times 0.1597 \times 0.0417 \times 0.3827$$
$$= 0.0255 + 0.00114 - 0.00501 = 0.20154 .$$
So, the intensity reflectance $R = r^2 = 0.02154 \approx 2.2\%$.

For the 700 nm wavelength, the optical thickness of 275 nm represents $275/700 = 0.3929$ of a wavelength, which is $0.3929 \times 2\pi$ radians phase change. This is equivalent to 141.4°. The vector diagram is now as shown in figure 9.8. Using the cosine rule,

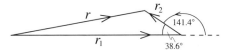

Fig. 9.8

$$r^2 = r_1{}^2 + r_2{}^2 - 2 r_1 r_2 \cos 38.6°$$
$$= (0.1597)^2 + (0.0417)^2 - 2 \times 0.1597 \times 0.0417 \times 0.7815$$
$$= 0.0255 + 0.00114 - 0.0104 = 0.01624 .$$

So, the intensity reflectance $R = r^2 = 0.01624 \approx 1.6\%$.

The reflectances at one surface with a single layer film are:

Wavelength	Reflectance
400 nm	2.2%
550 nm	1.4%
700 nm	1.6% .

---

11   Explain the use of the strain tester for examining heat-toughened glass spectacle lenses.

The strain tester (or polariscope) consists of a source of unpolarised white light which illuminates a sheet of polarising material. The light crosses a space of perhaps 5 cm and meets the analyser, a sheet of polarising material with its transmission axis perpendicular to that of the polariser (the first sheet). A lens which has been heat-toughened is placed in the space between the polariser and the analyser. Where the direction of stress in the compression layer (in and near the surfaces) is parallel or perpendicular to the polariser's transmission axis, no light emerges from the analyser. This results in the typical strain patterns for plus and minus lenses where the black regions are referred to as Maltese crosses in figure 9.9. Elsewhere, the electric vectors have been rotated and are no longer perpendicular to the analyser's transmission axis. Hence, some light passes through the system over these regions of the lens. Since an untoughened lens is not subject to stress, except where a frame rim presses unduly upon it, no light emerges when such a lens is placed in the strain tester so the instrument allows the dispenser to verify that lenses have been heat toughened, and conform to the order.

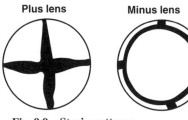

Plus lens   Minus lens

Fig. 9.9   Strain patterns.

10 OBLIQUELY CROSSED CYLINDERS

1 The following thin plano-cylinders are placed in contact:
plano / +2.50 x 80° and plano / +1.50 x 40°.
Determine, by a graphical method, the prescription of the resultant sph/cyl.

There are several graphical solutions to the problem of obliquely crossed cylinders, but the best known and easiest to use is often referred to as *Stokes' Construction*. This is similar to the parallelogram of forces, except that the angles are doubled. The construction is simplified if both cylinders are positive (or negative). All angles are measured anticlockwise and are taken to be positive. The symbols are as follows:
F_1 and F_2 are the two cylinder powers two be combined.
α is the angle between the two cylinder axes (both cylinders expressed with the same sign).
C is the resultant cylinder power found when the lenses are placed in contact.
2θ is the angle between the axes of F_1 and the resultant cylinder C.
S is the resultant sphere power.

1 If necessary, transpose the plano cylinders so that both are positive. (NB. Any spheres arising as a consequence of this will have to be taken into account in the final step.)
2 Select the cylinder whose axis is numerically closer to zero and call this cylinder F_1.
3 Using a convenient scale, construct F_1 along its axis direction.
4 Construct F_2 to scale at the angle 2α from F_1; that is, twice the difference between the two axes.
5 Complete the triangle by joining F_2 to the origin. This gives the magnitude of the resultant cylinder power C. (C will be positive if F_1 and F_2 are positive.)
6 Measure the angle between F_1 and C. This is 2θ. To express the resultant cylinder's axis in standard notation, θ must be added to the axis of F_1.
7 Find the sphere from
$$S = \tfrac{1}{2}(F_1 + F_2 - C).$$
8 Add to S any sphere resulting from step 1.

Fig. 10.1

Scale 1 inch : 1 D

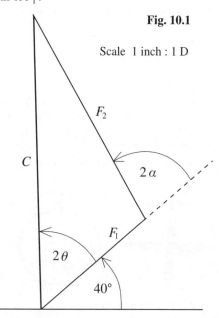

Using this method, the following graphical construction for the resolution of the obliquely crossed cylinders can be obtained. In this problem, $F_1 = +1.50$ x 40° and $\alpha = 40°$, so $2\alpha = 80°$. In figure 10.1, the scale used is 1 inch $\equiv$ 1 D of cylinder power.

By measurement, the resultant cylinder is $C = 3.13$ D and $2\theta = 52°$.

Therefore, $\theta = 26°$. Adding the axis of F_1, the axis of the resultant cylinder is $26° + 40° = 66°$.

128

The sphere is $S = \frac{1}{2}(F_1 + F_2 - C) = \frac{1}{2}(1.5 + 2.5 - 3.13) = +0.45$ D.

Hence, the resultant sph/cyl is $+0.45 / +3.1 \times 66°$.

The triangle in figure 10.1 can be used to find C and θ trigonometrically using the solutions:

$$\tan 2\theta = \frac{F_2 \sin 2\alpha}{F_1 + F_2 \cos 2\alpha} \quad \text{and} \quad C = \sqrt{F_1^2 + F_2^2 + 2F_1F_2 \cos 2\alpha} .$$

Thus, $\tan 2\theta = \dfrac{F_2 \sin 2\alpha}{F_1 + F_2 \cos 2\alpha} = \dfrac{2.5 \sin 80°}{1.5 + 2.5 \cos 80°} = 1.2729$, giving $2\theta = 51.8° \approx 52°$.

Then, $C = \sqrt{F_1^2 + F_2^2 + 2F_1F_2 \cos 2\alpha} = \sqrt{1.5^2 + 2.5^2 + 2 \times 1.5 \times 2.5 \cos 80°} = 3.13$.

The axis of C and the sphere power S are then calculated as before.

---

2   **What is the sph/cyl equivalent of the following pair of obliquely crossed thin cylinders?**
       plano / –2.00 x 90° and plano / –3.00 x 45°.

Method 1 — using minus cylinders

Using the rules set out in question 10.1, figure 10.2(a) shows the construction with $F_1 = -3$ and $F_2 = -2$. $\alpha = 45°$, so $2\alpha = 90°$. By measurement, the resultant cylinder is

     $C = -3.6$ D and $2\theta = 34°$.

Adding the axis of $\theta = 17°$ to $F_1 = 45°$ gives the axis of the resultant cylinder. That is,

     $\theta + F_1 = 17° + 45° = 62°$.

The sphere is

     $S = \frac{1}{2}(F_1 + F_2 - C)$

        $= \frac{1}{2}[(-3) + (-2) - (-3.13)]$

        $= -0.7$ D.

The resultant sph/cyl is therefore

   -0.7 DS $/ -3.6$ DC $\times 62°$.

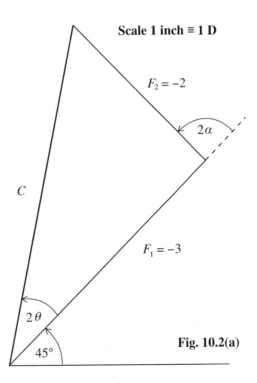

Scale 1 inch ≡ 1 D

$F_2 = -2$

2α

C

$F_1 = -3$

2θ

$45°$

Fig. 10.2(a)

Method 2 — using plus cylinders

Using Stokes' Construction, as set out in question 10.1, it can be seen that step 1 applies since both cylinders are negative. Transposing each cylinder gives

$$-2.00 \, / +2.00 \text{ x } 180 \quad \text{and} \quad -3.00 \, / +3.00 \text{ x } 135.$$

Hence, the sphere power thus arising must be taken into account at the end of the calculation. The cylinders which are being combined are therefore

$$\text{plano} \, / +2.00 \text{ x } 180 \quad \text{and} \quad \text{plano} \, / +3.00 \text{ x } 135.$$

Two important points arise in this question. Firstly, the axis of one cylinder is 180° (see step 2 in question 10.1). Therefore this is the cylinder to be regarded as F_1, since $180° \equiv 0°$ in standard notation. Secondly, 2α is greater than 180°, but this poses no problems as long as the procedure is followed meticulously. Hence, $F_1 = +2.00$ x 180°, $\alpha = 135°$, so $2\alpha = 270°$.

By measurement from figure 10.2(b), $C = +3.6$ D, $2\theta = 304°$, so that $\theta = 152°$.

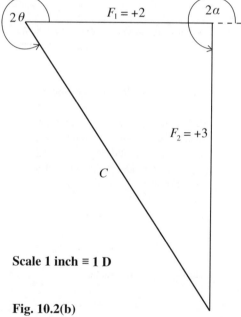

In this case, since the axis of F_1 is zero, there is nothing to add in order to state the axis of the resultant cylinder in standard notation. The sphere from the combined cylinders is

$$S = \tfrac{1}{2}(F_1 + F_2 - C)$$
$$= \tfrac{1}{2}[(+2) + (+3) - (+3.6)]$$
$$= +0.7 \text{ D}.$$

The spheres arising from the transposition must now be added:

$$(+0.7) + (-2.00) + (-3.00) = -4.3 \text{ D}$$

giving the final answer of

$$-4.3 \text{ DS} \, / +3.6 \text{ DC x } 152°.$$

Scale 1 inch ≡ 1 D

Fig. 10.2(b)

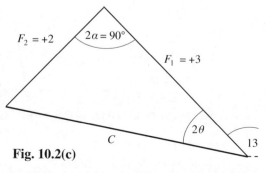

Incidentally, one could choose $F_1 = +3.00$ x 135° and $F_2 = +2.00$ x 180°, so that $2\alpha = 2(180° - 135°) = 90°$, which gives us the diagram in figure 10.2(c). Calculation again gives us $2\theta = 33.7°$, or approximately 34° as before, and $C = 3.6$ D exactly. These can be verified simply because the triangle is right-angled.

Fig. 10.2(c)

3 What single thin lens must be placed in contact with the lens $-1.00 / -2.00$ x $60°$ in order to obtain a combined power of $-4.00 / +2.00$ x $120°$?

With this question, it is essential to consider carefully the procedure which must be adopted before any calculation is embarked upon. Using the thin lens addition equation, $F = F_1 + F_2$, where:

the combined power is $\quad F = -4.00 / +2.00$ x $120°$
the first lens power is $\quad F_1 = -1.00 / -2.00$ x $60°$
and the unknown lens is $\quad F_2$,

then

$$F_2 = F - F_1 = (-4.00 \text{ DS} / +2.00 \text{ DC x } 120°) - (-1.00 \text{ DS} / -2.00 \text{ DC x } 60°)$$
$$= -4.00 \text{ DS} / +2.00 \text{ DC x } 120° / +1.00 \text{ DS} / +2.00 \text{ DC x } 60°$$
$$= -3.00 \text{ DS} / +2.00 \text{ DC x } 120° / +2.00 \text{ DC x } 60°.$$

That is, the unknown lens is $-3.00 \text{ DS} / +2.00 \text{ DC x } 120° / +2.00 \text{ DC x } 60°$. These cylinders can now be combined by Stokes' Construction following the procedure set out in question 10.1. Taking $F_1 = +2.00$ x $60°$ and $\alpha = 60°$, so that $2\alpha = 120°$, and drawing the diagram to scale, measurement gives $C = +2.0$ D and $2\theta = 60°$. Hence, $\theta = 30°$. Note that the axis of F_1 must now be added, so the axis of the resultant cylinder in standard notation is $30° + 60° = 90°$.

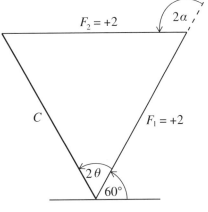

The sphere resulting from the addition of the obliquely crossed cylinders is

$$S = \tfrac{1}{2}(F_1 + F_2 - C)$$
$$= \tfrac{1}{2}[(+2) + (+2) - (+2)]$$
$$= +1 \text{ D}.$$

Fig. 10.3   **Scale 1 inch $\equiv$ 1 D**

The -3.00 D sphere must now be added to give $+1.00 + (-3.00) = -2.00$ DS, giving a final answer of $-2.00 \text{ DS} / +2.00 \text{ DC x } 90°$.

Alternatively, using the formulae for C and θ:

Then, $C = \sqrt{F_1^2 + F_2^2 + 2F_1 F_2 \cos 2\alpha} = \sqrt{2.0^2 + 2.0^2 + 2 \times 2.0 \times 2.0 \cos 120°} = 2.0 \text{ D}.$

and $\quad \tan 2\theta = \dfrac{F_2 \sin 2\alpha}{F_1 + F_2 \cos 2\alpha} = \dfrac{2.0 \sin 120°}{2.0 + 2.0 \cos 120°} = 1.7321$, giving $2\theta = 60°$.

The calculation for the axis of C and the resultant sphere follows as above.

4   A lens measure placed on a cylindrical surface reads +1.00 D. When rotated through 30° it reads +3.00 D. If neither position of the lens measure is along a principal meridian, find the power of the cylindrical surface.

Let the lens measure be at $\theta°$ to the cyl's axis meridian in the first setting, then using notional power relative to its axis meridian, where F is the cyl's power,

$$F \sin^2\theta = +1.00 \qquad (1).$$

After rotating the lens measure through 30°, we have $F \sin^2(\theta + 30°) = +3.00$ $\qquad$ (2).

Dividing equation (1) into equation (2) gives $\dfrac{\sin^2(\theta + 30°)}{\sin^2\theta} = \dfrac{+3.00}{+1.00} = 3$.

Taking the square root of each side and rearranging, $\sin(\theta + 30°) = \sqrt{3} \sin\theta$.

Expanding the LHS, $\sin\theta \cos 30° + \cos\theta \sin 30° = \sqrt{3} \sin\theta.$

Dividing both sides by $\sin\theta$, $\cos 30° + \cot\theta \sin 30° = \sqrt{3}$ $\qquad$ (3).

Now, $\cos 30° = \dfrac{\sqrt{3}}{2}$ and $\sin 30° = \dfrac{1}{2}$ so substituting these values into equation (3)

$$\frac{\sqrt{3}}{2} + \frac{1}{2} \cot\theta = \sqrt{3} \qquad \text{which rearranges to} \quad \cot\theta = 2\left(\sqrt{3} - \frac{\sqrt{3}}{2}\right) = \sqrt{3} .$$

Hence, $\theta = \text{arccot} \sqrt{3} = 30°$. Putting this value of θ in equation (1), rearranged to make F the subject of the equation, gives

$$F = \frac{+1.00}{\sin^2\theta} = \frac{+1.00}{\sin^2 30°} = \frac{+1.00}{(\frac{1}{2})^2} = +4.00. \qquad \text{That is, } F = +4.00 \text{ D.}$$

---

5   Two cylindrical lenses of like sign are crossed with an angle a between their axes. Find the meridians of the maximum and minimum powers of the resultant lens.

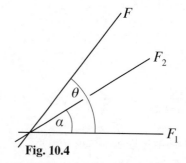
Fig. 10.4

The 'notional' power of a cylinder of power F along a meridian $\beta°$ to its power meridian is given by $F \cos^2\beta$ (see *Optics*, by Tunnacliffe and Hirst, Chapter 3). The notional power along θ due to the two crossed cyls F_1 and F_2 in figure 10.4 is therefore

$$F_1 \cos^2\theta + F_2 \cos^2(\theta - a) \qquad (1).$$

We can find θ for the maximum and minimum F by differentiating F with respect to θ since F is a function of θ for all θ. Then

132

$$\frac{dF}{d\theta} = 2F_1(-\sin\theta)\cos\theta + 2F_2(-\sin(\theta-\alpha))\cos(\theta-\alpha)$$

$$= -F_1\sin 2\theta - F_2\sin 2(\theta-\alpha) \qquad (2).$$

having used the trigonometrical identity $2\sin A\cos A = \sin 2A$.

Expanding the term $\sin 2(\theta - \alpha)$, using the identity $\sin(A - B) = \sin A\cos B - \cos A\sin B$, equation (2) becomes

$$\frac{dF}{d\theta} = -\{F_1\sin 2\theta + F_2(\sin 2\theta\cos 2\alpha - \cos 2\theta\sin 2\alpha)\}.$$

When this equals zero F has a local maximum or minimum value. That is, when

$$F_1\sin 2\theta + F_2\sin 2\theta\cos 2\alpha - F_2\cos 2\theta\sin 2\alpha = 0 .$$

Dividing both sides of this last equation by $\cos 2\theta$ gives

$$F_1\tan 2\theta + F_2\tan 2\theta\cos 2\alpha - F_2\sin 2\alpha = 0 .$$

which rearranges to give $\qquad \tan 2\theta = \dfrac{F_2\sin 2\alpha}{F_1 + F_2\cos 2\alpha} \qquad (3).$

Now, this equation will hold for $\tan 2\theta$, $\tan 2(\theta + 90°)$, $\tan 2(\theta + 180°)$ etc. The first and second solutions give the required meridians; that is, θ and $\theta + 90°$. When these values are placed in equation (1) the values of F_{max} and F_{min} are obtained. Note that θ is measured from the F_1 power meridian.

6(a) **Use equations (3) and (1) from question 5 above to find the sph/cyl resultant when a plano/+2.00 DC x 180° is placed in contact with a plano/+3.00 DC x 30°.**

  (b) **Solve the problem with a Stokes' Construction but solve the triangle with equations rather than a scale drawing.**

Part (a)
The powers of these cyls are along 90° and 120°. Using equation (3) from question 5 above, with $F_1 = +2.00$ x 180° $\equiv +2.00$ x 0°, $F_2 = +3.00$ x 30°, and $\alpha = 30°$,

$$\tan 2\theta = \frac{F_2\sin 2\alpha}{F_1 + F_2\cos 2\alpha} = \frac{3\sin 60°}{2 + 3\cos 60°} = 0.7423$$

whence $\theta = 18.29°$, measured from the F_1 power meridian (90°).

The maximum power lies along 18.29° relative to the power meridian of F_1, which places it along the 108.29° meridian. Now,

$$F_{max} = F_1\cos^2\theta + F_2\cos^2(\theta - \alpha) = 2\cos^2(18.29°) + 3\cos^2(18.29° - 30°)$$

$$= 1.803 + 2.876 = +4.68 \text{ D along } 108.29°.$$

133

Then, putting $\theta = 18.29° + 90° = 108.29°$,

$$F_{min} = F_1 \cos^2 \theta + F_2 \cos^2 (\theta - \alpha) = 2 \cos^2 (108.29°) + 3 \cos^2 (108.29° - 30°)$$

$$= 0.1969 + 0.1236 = +0.32 \text{ D along } 18.29°.$$

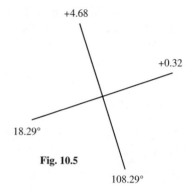

Fig. 10.5

Now, F_{min} is the sphere power and F_{max} is the sphere-plus-cyl power. The power diagram is shown in figure 10.5, from which the resultant sph/cyl is

$$+ 0.32 \text{ DS} / + 4.36 \text{ DC} \times 18.29°.$$

Part (b)

This method is really a simplified 'distillation' of the previous procedure. If we denote the resultant sphere and cylinder by S and C, respectively, it can be shown from figure 10.6 that

$$C = \sqrt{F_1^2 + F_2^2 + 2F_1 F_2 \cos 2\alpha}$$

or $\quad C = F_2 \dfrac{\sin 2\alpha}{\sin 2\theta}$ (1)

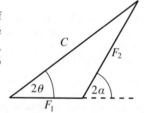

Fig. 10.6 $\quad 2\alpha = 60°$

which are obtained from the cosine rule and the sine rule applied to the triangle in figure 10.6. Also, $S = \frac{1}{2}(F_1 + F_2 - C)$ (2). Note that the F_1 and F_2 meridians here refer to the axes of the cylinders, but again $\tan 2\theta$ is

$$\tan 2\theta = \frac{F_2 \sin 2\alpha}{F_1 + F_2 \cos 2\alpha} = \frac{3 \sin 60°}{2 + 3 \cos 60°} = 0.7423$$

from which $\theta = 18.29°$. Here, this is the axis meridian of the resultant cylinder C.

Using the second of the equations in (1) to calculate the resultant cylinder C, with $F_1 = +2.00 \text{ DC} \times 180°$, $F_2 = +3.00 \text{ DC} \times 30°$ and $\alpha = 30°$, then

$$C = F_2 \frac{\sin 2\alpha}{\sin 2\theta} = 3 \times \frac{\sin (2 \times 30°)}{\sin (2 \times 18.29°)} = + 4.36 \text{ D}.$$

Hence, the resultant sphere is $S = \frac{1}{2}(F_1 + F_2 - C) = \frac{1}{2}(2 + 3 - 4.36) = +0.32 \text{ D}$ and the sph/cyl form is $+0.32 / +4.36 \times 18.29°$.

7   A patient has a   plano/+2.00 DC x 10°   prescription for one eye. It is dispensed as plano/+2.00 DC x 170° in error. Assuming each 0.50 D of uncorrected astigmatism blurs the patient's vision by one row of letters on the test chart, what will be the effect of the lens?

The patient would require a -2.00 DC x 170° to neutralise the wrong cyl, together with a $+2.00$ DC x 10° to provide the correct cyl. If we find the effect of these two cyls added together we will have found the single sph/cyl lens which should be added to the plano/+2.00 x 170° to correct the eye properly.

Transposing the -2.00 DC x 170, we have -2.00 DS / $+2.00$ DC x 80°. Bearing in mind this -2.00 DS, we add the $F_1 = +2.00$ DC x 10° to the $F_2 = +2.00$ DC x 80°, with $\alpha = 70°$ (that is, $\alpha = 80° - 10° = 70°$). The angle θ is found from

$$\tan 2\theta \ = \ \frac{F_2 \sin 2\alpha}{F_1 + F_2 \cos 2\alpha} \ = \ \frac{2 \sin 140°}{2 + 2 \cos 140°} \ = \ 2.7475 \ \Rightarrow \ \theta = 35.0°$$

The resultant cylinder C from adding these cylinders F_1 and F_2 is:

$$C \ = \ F_2 \frac{\sin 2\alpha}{\sin 2\theta} \ = \ 2 \times \frac{\sin (2 \times 70°)}{\sin (2 \times 35°)} \ = \ + 1.368 \text{ D}$$

The resultant sphere is $S = \frac{1}{2}(F_1 + F_2 - C) = \frac{1}{2}(2 + 2 - 1.368) = +1.316$ D, to which we must add the -2.00 DS we were bearing in mind earlier. Hence the total sphere is $-2.00 + (+1.316) = -0.684$ D. Hence, the lens which needs to be added to correct the error is -0.684 DS / $+1.368$ DC x $(10° + 35°) = -0.684$ DS / $+1.368$ DC x 45°.

The patient is 'uncorrected' by this amount of mixed astigmatism which is likely to blur back by 2 to 3 rows of letters on the test chart since the cyl required is between 1.00 D and 1.50 D.

Alternative method

In Tunnacliffe's *Introduction to Visual Optics* (1993 Edition, page 154), it is shown that the sphere, cyl and axis of the 'correcting' lens which needs adding is given by

$$(+ C \sin \beta) \text{ DS} / (-2 C \sin \beta) \text{ DC } x \ (45° + \theta + \beta/2)$$

where the axis α of the lens required to correct the focus is given by $\alpha = 45° + \theta + \beta/2$, θ is the correct axis and β is the error in the axis setting. Here then, $\theta = 10°$ and $\beta = 170° - 10° = 160°$. So, the correcting lens addition is

$$(+2) \sin 160° \text{ DS} / -2(+2) \sin 160° \text{ DC axis } (45° + 10° + 160°/2)$$

or $+0.684$ DS / -1.368 DC x 135° , which is the alternate sph/cyl form found earlier.

You should note that an off-axis cylinder in distance spectacles leaves the patient with mixed astigmatism where the disc of least confusion is on the retina.

8   What is the error involved when a prescription lens +4.00 DS / +3.00 DC is dispensed 5° off axis?

Using the alterntive method from question 7, the 'correcting' lens which needs adding is given by $(+C \sin \beta)\, \mathrm{DS} / (-2\, C \sin \beta)\, \mathrm{DC} \ \times\ (45° + \theta + \beta/2)$

where the axis α of the lens required to correct the focus is given by $\alpha = 45° + \theta + \beta/2$, θ is the correct axis and β is the error in the axis setting. Here then, θ is not stated so we leave it as it is, and $\beta = 5°$. So, the correcting lens to be added to the off-axis lens is

$$(+C \sin \beta)\, \mathrm{DS} / (-2\, C \sin \beta)\, \mathrm{DC} \ \times\ (45° + \theta + \beta/2)$$

$$=\ (+3) \sin 5°\, \mathrm{DS} / -2(+3) \sin 5°\, \mathrm{DC} \times\ (45° + \theta + 5°/2)$$

or $+0.26\, \mathrm{DS} / -0.52\, \mathrm{DC} \times 47.5°$.

---

9   A thin lens has a front surface power of +8.00 DS / +2.00 DC x 90°. What power must be worked on the back surface to produce a lens power of +4.00 DS / +1.00 DC x 40° ?

Let the thin lens power be $F = +4.00 / +1.00 \times 40°$ and the front surface power be $F_1 = +8.00 / +2.00 \times 90$. Then the back surface power F_2 is
$$F_2 = F - F_1 = (+4.00 / +1.00 \times 40°) - (+8.00 / +2.00 \times 90°)$$
giving $F_2 = -4.00 / +1.00 \times 40° / -2.00 \times 90°.$

Transposing the -2.00 DC x 90° to -2.00 DS / $+2.00$ DC x 180°, to make both cylinders have the same plus sign, we then require on the back surface

$$-6.00\, \mathrm{DS} / +1.00\, \mathrm{DC} \times 40° / +2.00\, \mathrm{DC} \times 180°.$$

Now, calling the cyls $F_1 = +2.00 \times 180°$ and $F_2 = +1.00 \times 40°$, and noting that these F_1 and F_2 symbols are not to be confused with the thin lens calculation earlier, we have the angle between the cyl axes is $\alpha = 40°$, and $2\alpha = 80°$, so for the resultant cyl's axis θ we have

$$\tan 2\theta\ =\ \frac{F_2 \sin 2\alpha}{F_1 + F_2 \cos 2\alpha}\ =\ \frac{1 \sin 80°}{2 + 1 \cos 80°}\ =\ \frac{0.9848}{2.1736}\ =\ 0.4531 .$$

from which $\theta = 12.19°$. This is the axis meridian of the resultant cylinder C since the axis of F_1, from which it is measured, is 180° (that is, 0°).

The resultant cylinder is $C = F_2 \dfrac{\sin 2\alpha}{\sin 2\theta}\ =\ 1 \times \dfrac{\sin (2 \times 40°)}{\sin (2 \times 12.19°)}\ =\ +2.39\, \mathrm{D}$.

Hence , the resultant sphere is $S = \tfrac{1}{2}(F_1 + F_2 - C) = \tfrac{1}{2}[(+2) + (+1) - (+2.39)] = +0.31\, \mathrm{D}.$

We must now add the -6.00 DS from the earlier stages to give the total sphere -5.69 DS.

The back surface must therefore have the power -5.69 DS / $+2.39$ DC x 12.19° or, in minus cyl form, -3.30 DS / -2.39 DC x 102.19° worked on it.

11   LENS FORM AND EFFECTIVITY

1   Explain what is meant by
   (a) nominal front surface power
   (b) vertex power allowance for the front surface.
   A +14.00 D meniscus is worked with a back surface power of −4.00 DS and an axial thickness of 9 mm. What power will the front surface have?

(a) In thin lens theory the power of the lens is equal to the sum of the surface powers; that is, $F = F_1 + F_2$. Since the lens is thin, the $BVP = F$. Or, in symbols, $F_v' = F$. Putting $F = F_v'$, we can write the thin lens equation as $F_v' = F_1 + F_2$ which rearranges to give $F_1 = F_v' − F_2$. When referred to thick lenses, this expression is called the *nominal front surface power* and is given the symbol F_{1N}. That is, $F_{1N} = F_v' − F_2$. The actual front surface power of a thick lens is then given by

$$F_1 = \frac{F_{1N}}{1 + \bar{t} F_{1N}} = \frac{F_v' − F_2}{1 + \bar{t}(F_v' − F_2)} .$$

(b) The vertex power allowance for the front surface is defined as $VPA_1 = F_1 − F_{1N}$.

Its purpose can be grasped more easily by looking at the equation in the form $F_1 = VPA_1 + F_{1N}$, from which it can be seen that, given a table of VPAs and for the centre thickness required and a simple calculation of F_{1N}, one can easily determine F_1, the actual power to be worked on the front surface of the lens in order to produce the required BVP. Nowadays, though, the whole calculation is done by computer!

In the problem, the nominal front surface power is $F_{1N} = F_v' − F_2 = (+14) − (−4) = +18$ D.

The actual front surface power is therefore

$$F_1 = \frac{F_{1N}}{1 + \bar{t} F_{1N}} = \frac{+18}{1 + 0.006 \times (+18)} = +16.25 \text{ D}$$

where $\bar{t} = \dfrac{t}{n} = \dfrac{0.009}{1.5} = 0.006$ m.

---

2   A lens of BVP +14.00 / −4.00 x 35 is made up in toric form with a +13.00 D base curve and in glass of refractive index 1.7 . The axial thickness is 8.5 mm. Find the powers of the cross curve and the sphere curve.

With this type of question, that is, with one of the two front surface powers given, it is necessary to step through the lens first to find the back surface power, and then step back to find the other front surface power. This particular lens is to be a front surface toric; that is, a plus base toric. By definition, the base curve of a toroidal surface is the power along the meridian of least curvature. This base curve must therefore correspond with the principal meridian of lower plus power. From the power diagram for this lens, it can be seen that this is the +10.00 meridian. The expression which gives the back surface power F_2, that is, the sphere curve, is

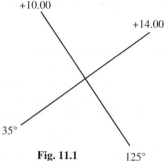

$$F_2 = F_v' - \frac{F_1}{1 - \bar{t}\,F_1}$$

which is derived from the back vertex power equation

and where $\quad \bar{t} = \dfrac{t}{n} = \dfrac{0.0085}{1.7} = 0.005$ m

in this case. Thus, the sphere curve (F_2) is

Fig. 11.1

$$F_2 = F_{v,125}' - \frac{F_{1,\text{base}}}{1 - \bar{t}\,F_{1,\text{base}}} = (+10) - \frac{(+13)}{1 - 0.005 \times (+13)} = -3.90 \text{ D}.$$

Stepping back to find the cross curve, we must use the other principal power; that is, $F_{v,35}'$.

Thus, $\quad F_{1,\text{cross}} = \dfrac{F_{v,35}' - F_2}{1 + \bar{t}\,(F_{v,35}' - F_2)} = \dfrac{(+14) - (-3.9)}{1 + 0.005 \times ((+14) - (-3.9))} = +16.43 \text{ D}.$

---

3 A meniscus lens made with $F_1 = +10.00$ D and $F_2 = -4.00$ D has centre thickness $t = 9$ mm and $n = 1.5$.

(a) What thin lens placed in contact with the convex surface will neutralise the meniscus?

(b) What would be the reading on a focimeter if the lens is placed (i) with its front surface on the lens rest, (ii) with its back surface on the lens rest?

(c) What would be the power of the front surface of the meniscus for the *BVP* to be zero? In this case, what would be the angular magnification of a distant object seen through the lens?

(a) The power of the thin neutralising lens must be equal in magnitude to the *FVP*, but opposite in sign. Noting that the reduced thickness of the lens is $\bar{t} = t/n = 0.009/1.5 = 0.006$ m, the *FVP* of the lens is

$$F_v = \frac{F_1 + F_2 - \bar{t}\,F_1 F_2}{1 - \bar{t}\,F_2} = \frac{(+10) + (-4) - 0.006 \times (+10) \times (-4)}{1 - 0.006 \times (-4)} = +6.09 \text{ D}.$$

Hence, the neutralising lens is −6.09 D.

(b) The reading on the focimeter with the front surface on the lens rest will be the *FVP* = +6.09 D. When the back surface is placed on the lens rest the reading is the *BVP*, F_v'.

That is; $\quad F_v' = \dfrac{F_1 + F_2 - \bar{t}\,F_1 F_2}{1 - \bar{t}\,F_1} = \dfrac{(+10) + (-4) - 0.006 \times (+10) \times (-4)}{1 - 0.006 \times (+10)} = +6.64 \text{ D}.$

(c) If F_v' is to be zero we have

$$F_1 = \frac{F_v' - F_2}{1 + \bar{t}\,(F_v' - F_2)} = \frac{0 - (-4)}{1 + 0.006 \times (0 - (-4))} = +3.91 \text{ D}.$$

The angular magnification through this afocal lens can be shown to be given by the *Shape Factor (SF)*. That is,

$$SF = \frac{1}{1 - tF_1} = \frac{1}{1 - 0.006 \times (+3.91)} = 1.024 \equiv 2.4\% \text{ increase in image size.}$$

---

4 **A trial lens of $BVP = +10.00$ DS was placed 12 mm from the eye during refraction. The spectacle lens supplied had a front vertex power of +9.75 D with a back surface power of –3.00 DS, centre thickness of 6 mm and a refractive index of 1.5. It had the same effectivity as the trial lens. What was the vertex distance?**

We need to find the effectivity (F_x) of the lens at the corneal vertex, where F_x may be called the corneal vertex refraction of the eye, the power of the front surface of the lens, and then the new vertex distance.

Hence, $F_x = \dfrac{F'_v}{1 - dF'_v} = \dfrac{+10}{1 - 0.012 \times (+10)} = +11.36 \text{ D.}$

The front surface power of the spectacle lens can be found by rearranging the expression for the front vertex power to give

$$F_1 = F_v - \frac{F_2}{1 - tF_2} = (+9.75) - \frac{(-3)}{1 - 0.004 \times (-3)} = +12.71 \text{ D},$$

where $t = \dfrac{t}{n} = \dfrac{0.006}{1.5} = 0.004 \text{ m.}$

Now, knowing the front surface power F_1, we can find the back vertex power:

$$F'_v = \frac{F_1 + F_2 - t F_1 F_2}{1 - t F_1} = \frac{(+12.71) + (-3) - 0.004 \times (+12.71) \times (-3)}{1 - 0.006 \times (+12.71)} = +10.39 \text{ D.}$$

Then $f'_v = \dfrac{1}{F'_v} = \dfrac{1}{+10.39} = +0.0962 \text{ m}$ and $f'_x = \dfrac{1}{F_x} = \dfrac{1}{+11.36} = +0.0880 \text{ m},$

so from figure 11.2 the vertex distance is $d = f'_v - f'_x = 0.0962 - 0.0880 = 0.0082 \text{ m} = 8.2 \text{ mm.}$

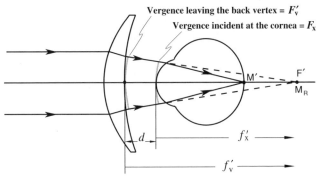

Vergence leaving the back vertex = F'_v

Vergence incident at the cornea = F_x

Fig. 11.2 $d = f'_v - f'_x$

5 What is the centre thickness of a plastic meniscus lens, $n_p = 1.560$, which has $BVP = +9.00$ D, $F_1 = +12.00$, and $F_2 = -4.00$ D?

As shown in figure 11.3, we can use the relationship

$$t = f_1' - f_{1N}' \quad \text{where } f_1' = \frac{n_1'}{F_1}, \ f_{1N}' = \frac{n_1'}{F_{1N}} \quad \text{and} \quad F_{1N} = F_v' - F_2.$$

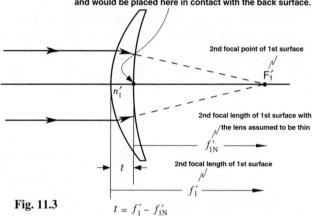

If the lens were thin, the front surface power would be F_{1N} and would be placed here in contact with the back surface.

2nd focal point of 1st surface

F_1'

n_1'

2nd focal length of 1st surface with the lens assumed to be thin

f_{1N}'

2nd focal length of 1st surface

f_1'

t

Fig. 11.3

$t = f_1' - f_{1N}'$

Note that n_1' is to the right of the first surface and is therefore equal to $n_p = 1.537$.

Hence, $f_1' = \dfrac{n_1'}{F_1} = \dfrac{1.560}{+12} = +0.1300$ m $= +130.0$ mm.

Then, $F_{1N} = F_v' - F_2 = (+9.00) - (-4.00) = +13.00$ D.

So, $f_{1N}' = \dfrac{n_1'}{F_{1N}} = \dfrac{1.560}{+13.00} = +0.1200$ m $= +120.0$ mm.

Therefore $t = f_1' - f_{1N}' = 130.0 - 120.0 = 10.0$ mm.

6   An eye is corrected for distance by a lens of BVP +9.50 DS. The distance from the back vertex of the lens to the cornea is 11 mm. What is the back vertex power of the lens required to correct the eye when the vertex distance is   (a) 7 mm   (b) 15 mm? (c) Compare your answers with the result of the approximate equation for the change in

power $\Delta F = \dfrac{-\Delta d\,F^2}{1000}$ where Δd is the change in vertex distance in mm, positive for an increase and negative for a decrease in d.

We shall use the equation $F_n = \dfrac{F_o}{1 + (d_n - d_o)F_o}$

where F_o is the original lens power at the original vertex distance d_o
and F_n is the new lens power at the new vertex distance d_n.

(a) The distances must be in metres, so $d_o = 0.011$ m and $d_n = 0.007$ m, then

$$F_n = \frac{F_o}{1 + (d_n - d_o)F_o} = \frac{+9.50}{1 + (0.007 - 0.011) \times (+9.50)} = +9.88 \text{ D.}$$

In practice, we would choose the nearest 0.25 D lower plus value; that is, +9.75 D.

(b) When $d_n = 0.015$ m, we have

$$F_n = \frac{F_o}{1 + (d_n - d_o)F_o} = \frac{+9.50}{1 + (0.015 - 0.011) \times (+9.50)} = +9.15 \text{ D.}$$

Here, we would choose to order +9.00 D.

(c) Using the approximate relationship with a decrease of 4 mm ($\Delta d = -4$ mm) in the vertex distance, we obtain

$$\Delta F = \frac{-\Delta d\,F^2}{1000} = \frac{-(-4) \times (+9.50)^2}{1000} = +0.36 \text{ D.}$$

So, the new lens power is $F_n = F_o + \Delta F = (+9.50) + (+0.36) = +9.86$ D, close enough to the exact +9.88 value obtained in (a).

Similarly, for the increase in vertex distance of 4 mm ($\Delta d = +4$ mm),

$$\Delta F = \frac{-\Delta d\,F^2}{1000} = \frac{-(+4) \times (+9.50)^2}{1000} = -0.36 \text{ D}$$

and the new lens power is $F_n = F_o + \Delta F = (+9.50) + (-0.36) = +9.14$ D, close to the +9.15 D found in (b).

In practice, we would use a set of tables which are calculated from the exact equation.

12 BEST FORM LENSES

1 List the five monochromatic aberrations and state their significance in the design of best form lenses (corrected curve lenses).

The five monochromatic aberrations are:

spherical aberration, coma, oblique astigmatism, field curvature, and distortion.

Spherical aberration and coma are image degrading aberrations dependent on the aperture of the lens stop. In the case of a spectacle lens, the pupil of the eye limits the diameter of the pencil of rays to such an extent that these aberrations may be neglected.

Oblique astigmatism, an image degrading aberration also, can be removed or reduced in a large range of spectacle lens powers when used in conjuction with a small diameter aperture stop. This is achieved by making the lens in the best form (shape) so that the oblique astigmatism introduced at the first surface is partially or wholly neutralised by that of the second surface. Modern lenses may additionally use the astigmatic properties of an aspherical surface to aid this neutralisation of oblique astigmatism.

A thin lens has a Petzval surface of radius $-nf'$, where n is the refractive index of the lens and f' is its focal length. When the eye rotates, its far point traces a spherical surface with its centre at the centre of rotation of the eye. Ideally, the Petzval surface of the correcting lens should coincide with the locus of the far point, the Far Point Sphere (FPS). If this were so, then oblique rays passing through the lens from a point object would focus on the FPS and, after refraction by the eye, would produce a 'point' image on the macula when the eye turned to look at the distant point object. In most cases, however, the Petzval surface is flatter than the FPS.

Distortion, an image deforming aberration, cannot be entirely removed from spectacle lenses. However, it is less pronounced in curved lenses than in flat lenses.

---

2 Explain what is meant by *far point sphere* and *vertex sphere*.

Far Point Sphere

Figures 12.1 and 12.2 show the far point sphere (FPS) for a hypermetropic and a myopic eye, respectively. M_R is the far point, F' is the second focal point of the spectacle lens, and R is the eye's centre of rotation. s is the fitting distance.*

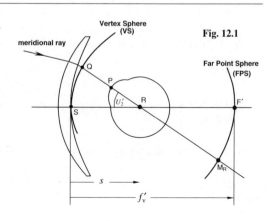

Fig. 12.1

* See *Introduction to Visual Optics*, section 3.21, for more detail.

In order that a sharp image of a point object is produced at the centre of the macula, the image formed by a spectacle lens must be at the far point of the eye. As the eye rotates about R, its centre of rotation, the far point moves over the imaginary spherical surface called the Far Point Sphere, which has radius M_RR and centre R, as shown in figures 12.1 and 12.2.

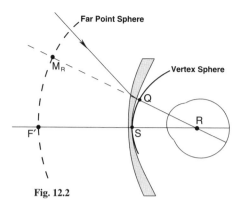

The Vertex Sphere

Fig. 12.2

Figures 12.1 and 12.2 also show the vertex sphere (VS). The vertex sphere has its centre of curvature at R and passes through the back vertex of the spectacle lens. In these diagrams, the back vertex of the spectacle lens is shown at the spectacle point S. The distance QM_R from the vertex sphere to the far point sphere is equal to the back vertex focal length (f_v') of the spectacle lens.

The purpose of the far point and vertex spheres is to allow comparison between the axial and oblique performances of the spectacle lens. Ideally, the vergence measured at the point Q for oblique gaze should equal that emerging from the lens at S in axial gaze.

---

3   **With the aid of diagrams, demonstrate the requirements of Point Focal and Percival best form lenses for distance vision.**

Point Focal Lenses

A narrow pencil of rays from a distant off-axis point object, limited by the eye pupil, should form a point image on the far point sphere; see figures 12.3(a) and (b). When calculating the oblique astigmatism using Coddington's Equations, the rays are infinitesimally close to the chief ray (the ray in the centre of the pencil of rays) so that the stop is effectively infinitesimally small in diameter! This is similar to the effect of paraxial ray calculations with reference to the principal axis and an axial point object.

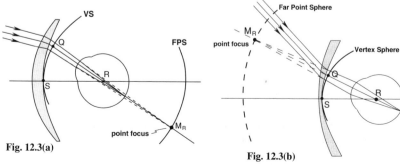

Fig. 12.3(a)

Fig. 12.3(b)

143

Percival Lenses

This lens design allows a small amount of oblique astigmatism but the tangential and sagittal image focal lines at F_T' and F_S' are made to straddle the FPS with the disc of least confusion on the FPS when

$$\frac{F_T + F_S}{2} = F_v' \qquad (1)$$

where F_v' is the back vertex power of the lens, F_T is the tangential oblique vertex sphere power, and F_S is the sagittal oblique vertex sphere power. With the aid of figure 12.4 we have the following definitions:

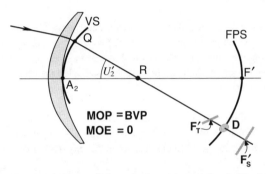

Fig. 12.4 The disc of least confusion (D) on the far point sphere (a Percival design).

Back Vertex Power of the lens $\qquad\qquad F_v' = \dfrac{1}{A_2 F'}$

Tangential Oblique Vertex Sphere Power $\quad F_T = \dfrac{1}{Q F_T'}$

Sagittal Oblique Vertex Sphere Power $\quad F_S = \dfrac{1}{Q F_S'}$

Oblique Astigmatic Error $\qquad\qquad\qquad OAE = F_T - F_S$

Mean Oblique Power $\qquad\qquad\qquad\quad MOP = \dfrac{F_T + F_S}{2}$

Mean Oblique Error $\qquad\qquad MOE = MOP - BVP = \tfrac{1}{2}(F_T + F_S) - F_v'$.

A zero MOE, $\tfrac{1}{2}(F_T + F_S) - F_v' = 0$, satisfies equation (1) and places the disc of least confusion on the far point sphere by refraction at the lens. If the Oblique Astigmatic Error is agreeably small for an ocular rotation of $U_2' = 35°$, say, then for practical purposes the lens may appear free from oblique astigmatism.

Percival lenses are flatter than point focal lenses, and this makes them appear neater. They also approximate well to near vision best form. Adopting the Percival principle also increases the range of BVPs which can be made in best form spherics. Roughly, this extends from −25 D to +10 D for refractive index 1.523 and from about −33 D to +11 D for refractive index 1.7.

Both point focal and Percival design principles can be applied to aspheric lenses, so the range of powers which can be made in best form is no longer limited as quoted above for spheric lenses (lenses without an aspherical surface).

---

4   Explain the role of pantoscopic tilt in spectacle fitting.

Generally, frames are fitted with the bottom rim tilted in about 10° with respect to the face plane. This prevents the patient from looking beneath the lower rim of the lens. This tilt also produces larger vertical components of the reaction forces acting on the fixed pads or the nasal rims of the frame thus more easily equilibrating that part of the frame's weight acting on the nose. To satisfy a lens design criterion, this fitting tilt requires that the vertical positioning of the optical centres must be chosen so that the optical axis of the lens passes through the eye's centre of rotation; see figure 12.5.

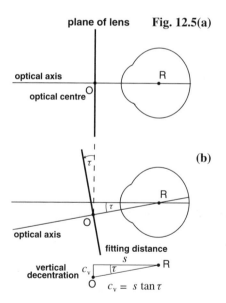

plane of lens   Fig. 12.5(a)

optical axis

optical centre O

R

(b)

optical axis

fitting distance

vertical decentration

$c_v = s \tan \tau$

When designing a lens, the optical axis is taken to pass through the eye's centre of rotation; see figure 12.5 (a).

Referring to figure 12.5(b), when the lens is fitted with a pantoscopic tilt, as is the usual practice, the relationship between the panto-scopic tilt (τ) and the vertical centration of spectacle lens can be shown to be: *for each 1° of tilt as shown, the optical centre should be moved 0.5 mm downwards from the pupil centre position* in the upper part of the diagram, ensuring the optical axis passes through R.

For snooker spectacles the pantoscopic tilt is in the other direction, so the optical centre must be placed above the pupil centre position accordingly. With adjustable pads, the frontal angle is adjustable independent of the plane of the front so that the pantoscopic tilt can be chosen from optical considerations alone.

5   A lens of BVP +8.00 DS has an oblique astigmatic error of +1.75 D and a mean oblique error of +1.00 D for the 30° zone of the lens. What are the oblique vertex sphere powers?

Notes: Tangential Oblique Vertex Sphere Power symbol is F_T

Sagittal Oblique Vertex Sphere Power symbol is F_S

Oblique Astigmatic Error	$OAE = F_T - F_S$
Mean Oblique Power	$MOP = \frac{1}{2}(F_T + F_S)$
Mean Oblique Error	$MOE = MOP - BVP = \frac{1}{2}(F_T + F_S) - F_v'$.

Using the expressions for MOE and OAE, we have

$MOE = \frac{1}{2}(F_T + F_S) - F_v'$ which rearranges to give

$F_T + F_S = 2(MOE + F_v') = 2 \times (1.00 + 8.00) = 18$,

that is, $F_T + F_S = 18$ (1).   Then, $OAE = F_T - F_S = 1.75$ (2).

Adding equations (1) and (2) gives $2F_T = 19.75$ D, $\Rightarrow F_T = +9.875$ D.

Then, from equation (1), $F_S = 18 - F_T = 18 - 9.875 = +8.125$ D.

That is, the tangential and sagittal oblique vertex sphere powers are +9.875 D and +8.125 D, respectively.

---

6   What are aspheric spectacle lenses and what are their advantages?

Aspheric spectacle lenses have one aspherical surface. In the early eighties it became possible to manufacture plastic aspherics reasonably cheaply. They were used to extend the best form range of high plus powers so that lenses for aphakia could have a reasonable oblique visual performance. More recently they have become available over the whole plus power range and even into the minus range.

The major advantages of aspheric lenses are:

(1)   Reduced centre thickness in plus lenses and reduced edge thickness in minus lenses.
(2)   Flatter lens form giving improved cosmesis.
(3)   Good oblique visual performance.
(4)   Distortion is reasonably controlled.
(5)   Reduced spectacle magnification (Shape Factor nearer unity) since the front surface is flatter.
(6)   Little sensitivity to fitting distance.

---

7   **What is meant by the 35° zone of a lens?**
Measured along the chief ray in the 35° zone of a plus lens, the distance from the back surface
to the vertex sphere is 4.55554 mm and the distances to the tangential and sagittal line foci are
179.34654 mm and 193.68147 mm, respectively. Calculate the OAE, the MOP and the BVP
of the lens if the $MOE = 0$. Assuming a distant object, what type of best form lens is this?

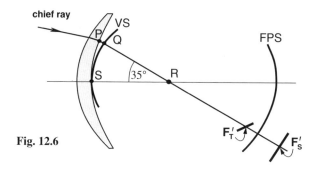

Fig. 12.6

The 35° zone measures that narrow zone of the lens where meridional rays are refracted with
35° ocular rotation. It is a way of stating that the ocular rotation is 35°.

Refer to figure 12.6 which shows the chief ray, the vertex sphere and the far point sphere.
The chief ray emerges from the back of the lens at the point P and intersects the vertex
sphere at Q. The tangential and sagittal focal lines are shown at F_T' and F_S', respectively.
Hence, with the distances in metres, the Tangential Oblique Vertex Sphere Power is:

$$F_T = \frac{1}{QF_T'} = \frac{1}{PF_T' - PQ} = \frac{1}{0.17934654 - 0.00455554} = +5.721 \text{ D.}$$

Similarly, the Sagittal Oblique Vertex Sphere Power is:

$$F_S = \frac{1}{QF_S'} = \frac{1}{PF_S' - PQ} = \frac{1}{0.19368147 - 0.00455554} = +5.287 \text{ D.}$$

The Oblique Astigmatic Error is:

$$OAE = F_T - F_S = (+5.721) - (+5.287) = +0.43 \text{ D} \text{ to two decimal places.}$$

The Mean Oblique Power is: $MOP = \frac{1}{2}(F_T + F_S) = \frac{1}{2}[(+5.721) + (+5.287)] = +5.50 \text{ D.}$

The BVP can be calculated from the definition of the Mean Oblique Error:

that is, $MOE = MOP - BVP$ which rearranges to give

$$BVP = MOP - MOE = (+5.50) - 0.00 = +5.50 \text{ D.}$$

A lens with zero MOE is a Percival lens.

8   An eye using a +6.00 point focal lens encounters a Mean Oblique Error (MOE) of −0.40 D in the 30° zone of the lens. If the diameter of the refracted pencil at the vertex sphere is 3 mm, what is the diameter of the blur disc on the far point sphere (FPS)? Is this amount of undercorrection (0.40 D) at 30° significant in practice?

Figure 12.7 shows the geometry in which the figures ABP and CDP are taken to be similar (approximate) triangles.

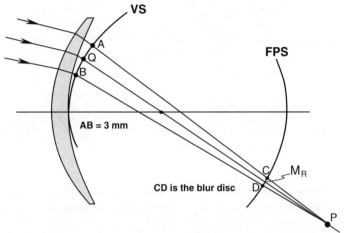

Fig. 12.7   The geometry for finding the blur disc diameter on the FPS

The distance from the vertex sphere to the far point sphere (QM_R) is equal to the back vertex focal length f_v' where

$$f_v' = \frac{1}{F_v'} = \frac{1}{+6.00} = +0.16666667 \text{ m} = +166.6667 \text{ mm}.$$

Since the Mean Oblique Error is $MOE = -0.40$ D, the Mean Oblique Power is

$$MOP = BVP + MOE = (+6.00) + (-0.40) = +5.60 \text{ D}.$$

The distance QP is given by $QP = \dfrac{1}{MOP} = \dfrac{1}{+5.60} = +0.1785714 \text{ m} = +178.5714 \text{ mm}.$

The blur disc diameter is the width of the refracted pencil as it crosses the far point sphere; that is, the distance CD. Then, by similar triangles,

$$\frac{CD}{M_RP} = \frac{AB}{QP} \Rightarrow CD = M_RP \times \frac{AB}{QP} = (QP - QM_R) \times \frac{AB}{QP}$$

$$= (178.5714 - 166.6667) \times \frac{3}{178.5714}$$

$$= 0.2000 \text{ mm}.$$

The undercorrection of 0.40 D in the 30° is of little consequence if the eye's depth of focus and accommodation are taken into account. Assuming a modest depth of focus of about 0.25 D, even without accommodation, this will reduce any perceived blur to a negligible amount. Further, one is not likely to maintain fixation at 30° for more than a second or two before the head is turned and the ocular rotation is reduced.

---

9 **What is the accepted principle of toric best form lens design?**
Below are the computer ray trace results for the lenses
    (a) +3.00 / +2.00 x 180 and (b) −5.00 / +2.00 x 180.
Which of the tyre or barrel forms of toroidal surface do you judge to be the better form for each lens? Explain your choices.

It is generally agreed that the oblique power, expressed as sph/cyl and measured at the vertex sphere as usual, should have equal cylinders in the base and cross curve meridian refractions. In the computations below, a difference of 0.02 D between oblique cyl powers is negligible.

(a) BVP = +3.00 DS / +2.00 DC. The ray traces below are for 30° ocular rotations on 60 mm diameter lenses, with a minumum edge thickness of 1 mm, and refractive index 1.5.

(i) Form   Plus Barrel, $F_2 = -5.00$ DS, $t = 5.93$ mm.
    Oblique Power   Along the base curve meridian   Along the cross curve meridian
                              +2.90 DS / +2.11 DC   +2.75 DS / +2.12 DC

(ii) Form   Plus Tyre, $F_2 = -6.50$ DS, $t = 6.19$ mm.
    Oblique Power   Along the base curve meridian   Along the cross curve meridian
                              +2.73 DS / +2.10 DC   +2.58 DS / +2.09 DC

(iii) Form   Minus Barrel, $F_2 = -5.50$ DB, $t = 6.00$ mm.   (DB = Dioptre Base)
    Oblique Power   Along the base curve meridian   Along the cross curve meridian
                              +2.58 DS / +2.22 DC   +2.65 DS / +2.22 DC

(iv) Form   Minus Tyre, $F_2 = -6.50$ DB, $t = 6.19$ mm.
    Oblique Power   Along the base curve meridian   Along the cross curve meridian
                              +2.73 DS / +2.10 DC   +2.58 DS / +2.09 DC

Answer
The two plus base forms have oblique cyl powers nearer the desired +2.00 DC of the BVP. Of the two plus base forms, the barrel toroidal surface has oblique sphere powers nearer the +3.00 required. Also, the sphere powers in the minus toroidal surface forms are relatively poor. Finally, the plus barrel form is the thinnest of the four lens forms.

(b) BVP = −5.00 DS / +2.00 DC. The ray traces below are for 30° ocular rotations on a lens with a centre thickness of 1 mm, and refractive index 1.5.

(i) <u>Form</u>   Plus Barrel, $F_2 = -9.37$ DS.
     <u>Oblique Power</u>   Along the base curve meridian   Along the cross curve meridian
                          −4.77 DS / +2.13 DC   −4.93 DS / +2.14 DC

(ii) <u>Form</u>   Plus Tyre, $F_2 = -9.00$ DS.
      <u>Oblique Power</u>   Along the base curve meridian   Along the cross curve meridian
                           −4.83 DS / +2.15 DC   −4.97 DS / +2.14 DC

(iii) <u>Form</u>   Minus Barrel, $F_2 = -7.25$ DB.
       <u>Oblique Power</u>   Along the base curve meridian   Along the cross curve meridian
                            −5.01 DS / +2.01 DC   −4.75 DS / +1.99 DC

(iv) <u>Form</u>   Minus Tyre, $F_2 = -7.75$ DB.
      <u>Oblique Power</u>   Along the base curve meridian   Along the cross curve meridian
                           −4.92 DS / +1.98 DC   −4.75 DS / +2.00 DC

Answer
The two minus base forms have oblique cyl powers nearer the desired +2.00 DC of the BVP. Of the two minus base forms, the barrel toroidal surface oblique sphere powers marginally better than the tyre form and the lens will have a slightly thinner edge because the base curve is 0.50 D flatter.